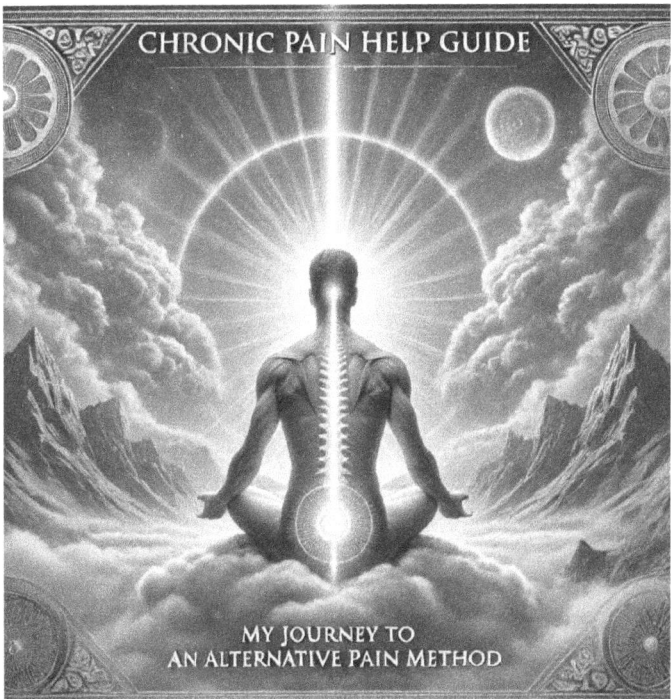

CHRONIC PAIN HELP GUIDE

MY JOURNEY TO
AN ALTERNATIVE PAIN METHOD

Second Edition

ISBN: 979-8-9923611-4-8

Published by Matthew K. Roberts

Winter Park, FL, United States

Cover design by Matthew K. Roberts,

Created with licensed elements from ChatGPT

Printed in the United States of America

This book is based on the personal experiences and opinions of the author. It is intended for informational purposes only and is not a substitute for professional medical advice, diagnosis, or treatment. Always seek the guidance of a qualified healthcare provider with any questions you may have regarding a medical condition.

FOREWORD

This book, "The Chronic Pain Help Guide: My Journey to an Alternative Pain Method," introduces a revolutionary, multi-step system designed to empower you to manage and ultimately remove muscle and nerve pain stemming from injuries throughout the body. Instead of enduring the persistent misery of a sore, dysfunctional back, this comprehensive method teaches you how to target pain at its source, often located in the spine and nervous system, and then systematically eliminate it. The core of this system is known as the Roberts Method, which employs a series of techniques called the Autonomic Bio Recovery Maneuvers (ABRM). The ability to remove chronic pain confers immense benefits, transforming daily life from one of debility to one of proactive management.

The Necessity of Innovation

My own necessity was the catalyst for this discovery. I suffer from arthritis in two discs in my back, a condition that was not only painful for years but profoundly debilitating. When the ABRM was first conceived, I had exhausted every conventional treatment option available to me. I had pursued spinal injections, routine massages, supportive braces, specialized exercises, rigorous stretching routines, and even back surgery. Despite these extensive efforts, I was left with persistent arthritis, spinal stenosis, debilitating memory issues, and residual neuropathy (nerve damage). If you have reached a point where chronic pain has consumed hours of your life, sending you on desperate searches for relief, then this alternative, neurological method is designed specifically for you. Beyond spinal discomfort, I have successfully applied the ABRM techniques to eliminate pain in joints, headaches, ankles, feet, knees, and, remarkably, even in areas connected to internal organs, such as the heart.

The Recovery Journey: Unwinding the Pain Cascade

This guide provides much more than just instructions on how to perform the maneuvers; it includes a raw and candid compilation of my own recovery journey from sometimes lifelong injuries and pains. Discovering the core ABRM technique was just the beginning; the real education started during the "recovery" journey that followed. I meticulously recorded my experiences, and after successfully managing the most severe, centralized pain in my back, I began to detect previously hidden pain in completely unrelated areas of my body. This process revealed a profound truth: the ABR Maneuvers do not just stop pain; they unwind a complex compensation cascade throughout the body. The method's effect on muscle groups, even in seemingly distant or unrelated body parts, demonstrated how interconnected the nervous and mechanical systems truly are.

Holistic Benefits: Mind and Body Recalibration

In addition to its pain-relieving properties, the Roberts Method offers significant neurological benefits that extend far beyond physical comfort. By calming and recalibrating the autonomic nervous system, the method can demonstrably enhance mental clarity and promote a far more positive mindset. The neurological influence of the ABRM can help reduce the persistent mental fog and depressive tendencies often linked to chronic pain. This comprehensive, two-pronged approach addresses both the physical discomfort and the cognitive and emotional aspects of well-being, establishing the ABRM as a powerful, holistic tool in your ultimate recovery journey. I sincerely hope that my shared experiences and the practical knowledge contained within this book will not only be helpful but paramount in your personal journey from chronic suffering to sustainable wellness.

Fun Fact: The placebo effect—a change in symptoms based purely on expectation—is so powerful in pain management because the brain releases its own natural pain-relieving chemicals, like endorphins, when it *anticipates* relief. This shows that the brain's belief system is intimately connected to the body's pain management circuitry.

DEDICATION

I give all glory to God for this book. It is by His grace, His guiding light, and His profound blessing that I was able to not only survive years of debilitating chronic pain but also carve out and discover this entirely new method for recovery. This discovery is a gift, and my greatest honor is sharing it with the world.

Next, and with all my heart, I dedicate this work to the absolute love of my life, my life partner and wife in every way that truly matters, Jacquelyn Albright (Jackie). Since 2002, Jackie, you have been my best friend, my greatest supporter, and the unshakable foundation of my life. For over two decades, we have shared everything: love, laughter, tears, and, most importantly, the joy of raising our two extraordinary sons, Matthew and Zachary. You bore witness to the darkest years of my pain, and your unwavering belief was the light that carried me through. This method exists because of your resilience alongside mine.

To my sons, Matthew and Zachary: Matt Matt and Zack, I love you deeply. You are strong, intelligent, loving, kind, and everything God blessed you to be. Your happiness and future were the constant, burning motivations that pushed me to find a way back to a healthy life.

I dedicate this book to my late parents, Ken and Jean Roberts. They raised me with a strong foundation of faith, unwavering morals, and an example of a devoted walk with God. They were always loving, fiercely supportive of my dreams, and they instilled in me the empathy and perseverance required for this work. I strive daily to emulate their positive attributes and miss them dearly.

Finally, I dedicate this book to my eldest brother and true American hero, Joseph Shane Crider. When his apartment building caught fire, Joseph's only thought was the safety of others; he selflessly saved everyone inside. Tragically, he became trapped, sustaining severe burns to over 60 percent of his body. He succumbed to his injuries just three short months later. He rests peacefully now at Arlington National Cemetery. Joseph, you are my hero, and your courage taught me the ultimate meaning of sacrifice and grit.

To my remaining seven brothers and sisters, as one of nine children, I send my love and prayers to you, your spouses, and your children. The countless great memories we share are treasures I cherish. We are an unbreakable family, and I carry each of you in my heart.

DISCLAIMER: READ BEFORE TRYING METHOD.

T he methods and maneuvers described in this book are designed to guide you on a transformative journey that could
significantly improve your life. This book is intended for individuals
who suffer from various forms of pain, including but not limited
to headaches, muscle pain, back pain, and other types of physical
discomfort, whether external or internal. The maneuvers I teach in
this manual are not meant to be combined with any other treatment,
including amateur or professional adjustments. This also includes any
added joint popping and/or cracking of the spine and/or any other
joint or bone in the body. The Roberts Method and Autonomic Bio
Recovery Maneuvers is a standalone technique. I would use extreme
caution when using massagers and even massage therapists. After us-

ing the Roberts method, the area will be tender. It is easy to re-injure the muscle.

Use at Your Own Risk: While applying this method to alleviate pain is straightforward in its explanation, it is equally important to understand that it can be physically challenging. The process involves targeting specific areas and injuries that cause pain. Additionally, bending and squatting are part of the steps to this method. This can be difficult if you lack mobility in your legs. For this reason, the Roberts method may not be suitable for everyone. While some aches and pains can be removed with a single application of the techniques, some injuries may require multiple applications to alleviate pain completely. I call this method a "pain journey" because after the pain is removed, it can seem like it may "travel" to a connected muscle or muscle group. What is really happening is your body is becoming aware of places that have been compensating for the original injury. I talk more about this concept in the chapter on muscle compensation. Pain caused by muscles, nerves, and joints is complex. The human body's response to pain is also complex. Sometimes, the pain or injury is so bad that the ABRM can only remove a small part of the pain at a time. The time it takes to remove pain altogether can vary. Sometimes, the pain is so intense that you must combine pressure with a specific position to achieve the desired effect.

The method presented in this book can be viewed as a skill that can be refined and improved over time. Eventually, you can target deep muscular pain that may require stimulating multiple points and even combining that with physical position with and/or without weights. Personally, I have been using my method for over a decade. During this time on my personal "recovery journey," I have improved my body's function on both the inside and outside. This method may give you the ability to maximize your potential for optimal health and wellness.

Medical Disclaimer: I am not a licensed medical professional nor do I have any formal medical training. This book is authored from a first-person perspective, rooted in my subjective experiences as an individual who has endured chronic and debilitating pain for many years. However, it is essential to note that I am no longer constrained by my pain, a change I attribute to the method outlined in this book.

This book provides readers with a technique for alleviating pain, restoring physical function, and enhancing their overall quality of life. While the methods and techniques presented are easy to understand, learn, and replicate, implementing the recovery process can be challenging. It may involve pain, require patience, and take time.

Broken Bones, diseases (acquired or born with), and elderly: Although I have used the techniques described in this book to alleviate pain from broken bones, such as a broken finger, this method will not repair or mend broken or damaged bones. The Roberts Method and Autonomic Bio Recovery Maneuvers (ABRM) can be used to remove pain associated with the fractured bone. However, it is not advised for many reasons. Broken bones are complex injuries. If the fracture is not reset and braced properly, it could result in more pain and even physical deformity.

I do not have experience working with any conditions other than my own, and as such, I can not and will not promise that I can help to manage and remove pain caused by acquired or diseases a person has been born with, such as Lyme's Disease, Parkinson's, and even Chronic pain conditions.

Persistence is Key: The road to recovery may not be easy, but perseverance is crucial. The techniques in this book are designed to empower you; however, the journey may require dedication and effort. Please continue with caution, and do not give up. By reading and using the information in this book, you acknowledge and accept the inherent risks involved and agree that the author shall not be held liable for any injury, harm, or loss resulting from applying the methods and techniques presented in this book.

THE BLUEPRINT FOR PAIN RELIEF: WHY YOU NEED THE THEORY BEFORE THE TECHNIQUE

H ave you ever tried a new therapy only to have the relief disappear as soon as you stopped the treatment? This book is designed to give you the power of permanence, structuring the journey in two essential parts to ensure you don't just temporarily manage pain, but fundamentally understand and correct its source. The Roberts Method is not a quick fix; it's a comprehensive neurological recalibration tool. Therefore, I highly recommend reading this book straight through, without skipping ahead. To effectively maximize the benefits of the Autonomic Bio Recovery Maneuvers (ABRM), a thorough understanding of the underlying theory is absolutely critical. This foundational knowledge will enable you to find the root of your pain faster, eliminate it more quickly and permanently, and gain a profound understanding of your body's intricate function.

Part One: The Theory and The Testimony

In the first section, I introduce the Roberts Method and the Autonomic Bio Recovery Maneuvers (ABRM). This part is devoted to explaining the *why* and the *how* of the therapy at a deep, neurological level.

Theoretical Foundations

Understanding the Blueprint: I will clearly explain the theoretical basis of the Roberts Method, detailing how it interacts directly with your body's electrical and mechanical systems.

The Body's Key Players: We will define the specific physiological components involved in this recovery process, focusing on the Autonomic Nervous System (ANS), the Central Nervous System (CNS), and the Articular Nervous System embedded in your joints. Understanding these parts explains how pain is created and how it moves.

Compensation Unmasked: I share crucial insights into how your body *compensates* for injury. Understanding this process will allow you to quickly trace symptoms (e.g., knee pain) back to their true, often distant, source (e.g., a spinal misalignment).

Compatibility and Context: A critical element of Part One is addressing the practical question of medication. I will clarify whether any medications are used alongside this therapy (Spoiler: The ABRM is non-chemical) and explain how this method complements or compares to other treatments, such as chiropractic adjustments, physical therapy, or traditional medical care.

The Personal Journey to Discovery

This part of the book is also where I share the raw, personal journey that necessitated this discovery. You'll read about the injuries and struggles I overcame, which serve as the case studies for the ABRM's effectiveness. This includes the story of my life-altering fall down the stairs at the age of fourteen, which herniated discs in my back, the compounding injuries to my knees and shoulders, and the eventual necessity of lower back surgery. Furthermore, I share honest accounts of other challenges I faced during my recovery, including battles with anxiety, depression, and addiction, illustrating how this physical method provides surprising neurological and psychological benefits that enhance mental clarity and promote a positive mindset.

Part Two: The Maneuvers and The Mastery

In the second section, the focus shifts entirely to practical application. This is your comprehensive manual for using the ABRM.

Step-by-Step Application

Simple Instructions: I provide detailed, step-by-step instructions on how to perform each of the Autonomic Bio Recovery Maneuvers. I break down every step into simple, easily understandable directives.

Expectation Management: I clarify exactly what to expect as you go through each phase of the method, including the sensations you will experience during pain removal. I also offer post-use guidance, explaining how you may feel immediately after a session and what signs indicate successful nerve recalibration.

Tools for Deeper Pain: I provide specific guidance on tools that can help you reach pain at its deepest source. This is crucial because if you cannot reach pain at its deepest source, you will not be able to fully remove it. Fortunately, no special equipment is required; the primary tools are often simple household items like a wall corner or a marker to track "pain points."

The Promise of Relief: I explain the timeline for relief and how to recognize when you have achieved the maximum possible benefit from the Roberts Method, guiding you toward a permanent, pain-managed state.

Fun Fact: Your body's fastest nerve signal, which carries the immediate, sharp pain of an injury, travels at speeds up to 268 miles per hour. This instant communication between your body and brain is one of the rapid electrical signals the ABR Maneuvers are designed to intentionally influence!

TABLE OF CONTENTS

C hronic Pain Help Guide: My Journey to an Alternative Pain Method

Copyright

Foreword

Dedication

Disclaimer: Read Before Trying Method.

How To Read This Book

Table of Contents

1.Part 1: Welcome to the ABR System: Are You Ready to Stop Searching for Relief?

2.Beyond Medication, Why the World Needs New Paths to Healing

3.My Story: From Childhood Fall to Spinal Crisis: My Journey to the ABR Method

Photo taken in 2015 after back surgery (Before method use)

10 years later. I still have arthritis and Spinal Stenosis.

4. The Electrical Blueprint: Pain, Posture, and the Autonomic Nervous System

5. The Central Command Center: Why Back Pain is Brain Pain

6. The Hidden Cost of Compensation & Why Your Body Lies to You

7. The Illusion of Movement & Why Pain Only Seems to Travel

8. The Unavoidable Slide: Can We Really Fight Age-Related Breakdown?

9. Part Two: Step 1: Finding Pain Points and The Three-Point Stimulation Technique

10. The Mechanics of Recalibration: Steps 2 Through 5 of the ABR Maneuvers

11. Tips to use the ABR Maneuvers more effectively. Removing Complex and Deep Muscle Pain. How to use positioning and weights to target and remove deep pain and hard-to-reach muscles pain; as well as joint related pain.

12. The Ground-Up Solution: Why Knee Pain Starts in Your Feet

13. The Body's Weakest Link: How Shoulder Pain Became a Roadmap to Healing

14. The Secret Language of Your Hands: Why They Hold Your Body's Stress

15. The Engine of Vitality: How to Command Your Heart and Lungs

16. Beyond Pain Relief: Why Exercise is the Anchor of the Roberts Method

17. Grit, Resilience, and the Relentless Pursuit of Healing

18.Empowered Healing: The Role of Self-Reliance and Self-Care in Pain Management

19.Beyond Pain: The Quiet Triumph of "Business as Usual"
Back Cover

CHAPTER ONE

PART 1: WELCOME TO THE ABR SYSTEM: ARE YOU READY TO STOP SEARCHING FOR RELIEF?

W elcome to the **Autonomic Bio Recovery (ABR) System** with the Roberts Method. If you are reading these words, chances are you are weary from years spent searching for an elusive solution to persistent, chronic pain—whether it resides in your back, shoulders, head, feet, arms, or hands. Perhaps you are dealing with discomfort in your knees or other major joints from an injury that simply refuses to resolve, or you might be grappling with chronic headaches, breathing difficulties, or issues like sleep apnea, which can be unexpectedly linked to dormant or underdeveloped muscles. I understand this frustration intimately. My name is Matthew Roberts, and though my name may not be widely known, that fact is irrelevant to your recovery. Like you, I faced significant physical devastation, suffering from chronic pain for over half my life due to compounding injuries and a debilitating condition called **spinal stenosis**. If you are tired of living in pain, exhausted by the endless online searches for relief, and frustrated by failed treatments—from stretches and injections to even surgery—then this book and this method are specifically for you.

From Debilitation to Discovery: The Origin Story

I decided to publish this book to share a remarkable, effective method that allowed me to fundamentally reclaim my life and resume the pursuit of my goals and dreams. The journey began tragically during my early teenage years with a severe work injury. While heading downstairs to retrieve items, I slipped, fell, and landed heavily on my back, resulting in **herniated discs** in both my upper and lower spine. This fall initiated a two-decade span of chronic, debilitating pain that severely limited my mobility. Even after undergoing back surgery, I experienced new, referred pain that left me at my lowest point, utterly convinced I would never be free from constant discomfort. Though deep depression followed, my faith in God remained my anchor. During a time of intense prayer and despair following my surgery,

I experienced a life-changing spiritual encounter. It was then that I was blessed with the insight and curiosity required to meticulously carve out and discover this gift that I now feel compelled to share with humanity. I am not a chiropractor or a doctor; I am simply an educated individual with profound faith, but the ABR System is a non-religious, physiological process unlike any other pain treatment available today.

Unpacking the Roberts Method: Structure and Tools

This book is logically structured into two comprehensive parts. **Part One** establishes the theoretical foundation of the ABR Method. I will explain the complex parts of the nervous system and body involved in the recovery process, detailing precisely how the body compensates for injuries and how these compensatory patterns affect long-term pain management. I will also provide a comparative analysis of the ABR System alongside other alternative treatments, such as chiropractic medicine, osteopathy, and even standard techniques like massage, clarifying how they relate to the ABRM. Throughout the first part, I share personal stories illustrating how I applied these techniques to my own devastating injuries and address potential challenges you may encounter. Though the ABRM can remove pain, it acknowledges that chronic conditions often involve multiple biological and neurological factors.

Part Two is a practical, step-by-step guide to performing the **Autonomic Bio Recovery Maneuvers**. I will explain the approach for each step and, crucially, help you recognize the precise moment a step has been successfully completed, enabling you to confidently move to the next. This method took over seven years to fully develop, but you can begin implementing these techniques as soon as you complete this book. The beauty of the ABR Maneuvers—also known as the Roberts Method—is that it is an independent, non-assisted, alternative pain management therapy designed to address muscle and nerve pain from a multitude of sources. You can complete every step on your own, significantly reducing your time spent recovering from injury and physical discomfort. Furthermore, no specialized equipment is required. I will show you how to utilize common household items—with the main "tool" being the **corner of a wall**—and a simple ink pen or marker to track "pain points." While these minimal tools are sufficient, I will also show you how to enhance the method using exercise equipment, massage balls, and even weights.

The Rippling Effect of Pain and Recovery

When you are injured, your body initiates a healing cascade, but its capacity to fully resolve complex, years-long issues independently is limited. Part of the healing process involves the systematic removal of pain, which is often accompanied by increased localized blood flow once nerve signals normalize. This is where the ABR Maneuvers become essential. Consider a shoulder injury: the damage doesn't stay confined to a single area. It creates an initial impact point, and then the pain **spreads or ripples outward**. Injuries to major, compound systems like the shoulders, knees, or core often trace back to one or more points in the spine and surrounding back muscles. You can and should trace the pain from the shoulder down the arm, looking for muscle tension and instability at every point of connective tissue, including the hands and fingers. Yes, chronic back injuries frequently affect hand strength and dexterity.

This intricate network of pain—where a single shoulder injury can generate widespread issues—highlights the complexity of the human body, but also the predictability of its repair. Just as a bruise heals from the outer edges inward to the center, the ABRM works by systematically addressing the widespread pain and tension placed on surrounding muscles, which is essential for successful injury recovery.

By reading my journey, you will gain a clearer understanding of the challenges you may encounter while using the Roberts Method. My aim in sharing this book is to provide individuals suffering from pain with a way to not only manage their discomfort but to fully recover and regain control of their lives, just as I have. **You can fight back!** You can take back control. If my journey and this method can inspire and aid even a single person, this book will have achieved its purpose.

Fun Fact: Despite what most people think, a herniated disc rarely pinches a nerve directly. Instead, the disc material leaks out and causes a powerful **inflammatory response** around the nerve root, and it is the **chemical irritation and swelling** that typically creates the most excruciating pain.

CHAPTER TWO

BEYOND MEDICATION, WHY THE WORLD NEEDS NEW PATHS TO HEALING

M odern medicine has achieved extraordinary and often life-saving advances, particularly in acute care, surgical techniques, and diagnostics. However, it continues to face persistent limitations when dealing with the complex, systemic nature of chronic pain. For many decades, the standard approach has been to prescribe medications such as painkillers, anti-inflammatories, muscle relaxers, and antidepressants—primarily to reduce the symptoms, rather than to invest in identifying or addressing the deeper, root causes of the suffering. This pharmaceutical reliance has left millions of people in a state of dependency, often without achieving satisfactory or long-term relief. While drugs have an essential and often lifesaving place, they are not designed to be universal solutions. When it comes to managing long-term, non-life-threatening chronic pain, they frequently treat the surface signals rather than the source of the mechanical or neurological dysfunction.

This systemic issue is not the fault of any single entity but is the result of an entire medical paradigm built on a reactive model. The focus prioritizes interventions that offer swift, albeit temporary, symptomatic relief over those that seek to restore function or correct underlying imbalances within the nervous system, muscles, joints, or posture. Most chronic pain medications operate by temporarily interrupting pain signals; they do not possess the capacity to teach the body how to heal, reposition, or effectively recalibrate its structural and neurological systems. They alter chemical pathways, such as blocking the transmission of neurotransmitters or reducing inflammation chemically, but they rarely help the nervous system to reorganize or correct the primary mechanical imbalances that initiate the pain signals in the first place. For numerous individuals, this creates a vicious and debilitating cycle: chronic pain leads to medication, medication leads to chemical tolerance or undesirable side effects, and increasing symptoms lead to stronger prescriptions, all while the original, structural cause of the pain remains fundamentally untouched. Meanwhile, the body's intrinsic ability to heal, adapt, and self-recalibration capability primarily managed by the nervous system—is often neglected or unsupported.

The opioid crisis stands as a stark and tragic illustration of the limitations inherent in this symptom-suppression model. The crisis did not emerge because patients simply sought dependency; it occurred because millions of individuals were suffering immensely, and the most heavily promoted and widely available tools focused exclusively on chemical relief rather than addressing the root causes of their pain. For decades, pain was viewed as a simple chemical imbalance that could be successfully muted with the correct pharmaceutical formula. Opioids were highly effective at this task, dramatically altering how the brain interpreted the pain signals. However, they accomplished nothing to correct the mechanical, neurological, or postural defects that initially produced the pain. As patients inevitably developed tolerance to the drug, dosages were increased, which led directly to dependency. This crisis revealed a profound truth: chemical relief is an inadequate long-term substitute for structural, neurological, or autonomic correction. Painkillers can silence the body's alarm system, but they possess no mechanism to repair the underlying electrical wiring or realign the compromised mechanical system. Most people who became dependent were not careless; they were desperate for any tool that quieted their suffering, and they were given a tool that disconnected them from their pain signals without guiding the body toward genuine, permanent recovery. This void is what holistic, nerve-based approaches are positioned to fill today.

The crucial point is that pharmaceutical treatments are not inherently harmful; they are incredibly valuable, essential tools for a specific range of problems, especially acute injuries, infections, or emergencies. The issue lies in the system's lack of accessible alternatives offered alongside medication. Patients deserve more options than solely pills or surgery; they need methods that genuinely complement medical care, not replace it, and approaches that empower the body's self-healing capabilities rather than suppressing its essential signals. The human body is not merely a machine with interchangeable parts; it is a holistic electrical, mechanical, chemical, and neurological system inextricably intertwined. Pain is multifaceted—it is not only a chemical signal that can be muted but is also a mechanical signal, an electrical signal, a postural warning, and an autonomic signal. The traditional model addresses only one of these vital dimensions.

The Autonomic Bio Recovery (ABR) Maneuvers are designed to step directly into the gap left by these traditional approaches. Instead of chemically interrupting pain, the ABR Maneuvers interact with the body's inherent electrical and neurological pathways. They specifically stimulate the autonomic nervous system and engage the sensory nerves embedded in the articular system (joints and ligaments), communicating with the central nervous system in a way that medication cannot replicate. This provides a natural, non-chemical methodology for reducing pain by guiding the body into systematically releasing long-standing compensation patterns rather than merely suppressing the symptoms those patterns generate. Holistic methods like ABR acknowledge that pain is a critical piece of information from the body's own intelligence, not an error to be silenced. When pain is followed, understood, and worked through layer by layer—as in this system—the body is given the opportunity to correct the underlying dysfunction itself.

This new era of healing demands methods that align with the body's natural processes. In contrast to the Western focus, Eastern medical traditions (such as Traditional Chinese Medicine and Ayurveda) have always recognized the body as an interconnected system where mechanical tension, nerve pathways, and what they term "energy flow" influence one another profoundly. For millennia, these traditions observed principles that align uncannily with modern neuromuscular theories: that pain moves along predictable pathways; that distant regions compensate for local tension; and that the nervous system holds memory of trauma. They recognized, long before advanced Western science, that the body communicates through electrical pathways, and that pain is often the body's language for expressing systemic imbalance.

The ABR Method uniquely sits at the crossroads of these two great medical paradigms. It acknowledges the scientific rigor of Western medicine, the electrical nature of pain, the function of the autonomic nervous system, and biomechanics—while simultaneously embodying the holistic, whole-body understanding of interconnectedness emphasized in Eastern traditions. The ABR Maneuvers are not mystical, but they deeply respect the body's internal intelligence. They are non-pharmaceutical, yet they exert powerful neurological effects. They are not purely structural, yet they profoundly influence posture, movement, and load distribution. They succeed because they harness what both traditions recognize in their own language: the body is fully capable of guiding its own healing when given the correct, specific stimulus. Western science tells us *how* the nerves work; Eastern wisdom teaches us *how* pain flows; the ABR method unifies these truths into a practical, accessible system that addresses the cause of pain, not merely its perception.

Fun Fact: The nociceptors, the specialized sensory nerves responsible for detecting potential damage, do not actually send a "pain" signal. They transmit a signal of potential threat to the brain. It is the brain's job to interpret that electrical signal, factoring in context, emotion, and previous experience, and then generate the *feeling* we call pain. This is why pain is often called an output of the brain, not an input from the tissues.

Fun Fact #2: The concept of phantom limb pain, where an amputee feels pain in a missing limb, is one of the clearest demonstrations that pain is an electrical and neurological event interpreted by the brain, not just a physical problem in the tissue. The pain is generated entirely within the nervous system's map.

CHAPTER THREE

MY STORY: FROM CHILDHOOD FALL TO SPINAL CRISIS: MY JOURNEY TO THE ABR METHOD

I n this chapter, I will not just recount a series of accidents; I will trace the physical devastation that became the unlikely foundation for a breakthrough. Every debilitating injury, every failed treatment, and every moment of despair ultimately guided me toward discovering an alternative pain management technique—the Autonomic Bio Recovery (ABR) Maneuvers—that conventional medicine never offered. My story began simply, filled with the typical joys of childhood: I spent countless hours playing sports like baseball and football with friends and family, and yes, plenty of video games, too. My brothers and sisters were my first best friends. Amidst the great times, we faced genuine struggles; money was often tight, which meant food resources were also limited. Yet, thanks to the immense effort and faith of my mother and father, and the divine provision we relied on, I never went hungry or went without my core needs being met. I thank my Mom and Dad for their sacrifice, and we all thank God most of all.

The Domino Effect of a Childhood Fall

The catastrophic event that derailed my physical health occurred when I was just fourteen. To help my family and to afford my own clothes and shoes, I took a job at a fast-food restaurant, perhaps too young for the responsibilities involved. One fateful day, while heading downstairs to retrieve more cups, the slippery stairs betrayed me. I slipped and fell hard, landing squarely on my back. My life changed forever in that instant. The fall resulted in herniated discs in both my upper and lower back. These injuries immediately triggered a profound domino effect, leading to pervasive muscle weakness and chronic, spreading pain that lasted for more than fifteen debilitating years. The process of reversing these negative, cumulative effects and damage has since required years of focused effort and dedication.

Compounding Traumas and the Road to Surgery

The initial trauma was compounded by subsequent, severe injuries that worsened my lower back condition. The first occurred in high school during a weightlifting accident while I was performing an incline squat. I heard a distinct pop in my lower spine. I strongly suspect that the underlying lower spinal weakness was a direct result of the initial upper back damage, demonstrating a chain reaction where the body compensates until a weak link finally breaks. For years, my upper and lower back were locked in constant agony. In 2009, I suffered a third major injury in a freak trampoline accident where my spine folded the opposite way, further herniating the already damaged disc in my lower back. The pain was immediate and excruciating, rendering me unable to walk. I was rushed to the hospital by ambulance. While a spinal injection temporarily restored my ability to walk, the structural damage and pain persisted. Despite this immense suffering, I clung to resilience, remaining active and engaging in sports and exercise, refusing to let the pain completely dictate my life.The Climax: Cauda Equina and Spinal Stenosis

The culmination of these traumas occurred in 2015 while I was hiking in Colorado. This final, severe injury stole not only my ability to walk but also my ability to stand. I was urgently told that surgery was necessary. The root of the problem was nerve root compression in my lower spine, which escalated into a serious condition known as Cauda Equina Syndrome. This resulted in a constellation of terrifying symptoms, including loss of sensation, muscle wasting, intense tingling (paresthesia) in my lower extremities, and even cognitive issues like brain fog and memory problems. I was also diagnosed with a degenerative spine disease called spinal stenosis. After waiting a week in the hospital due to the extreme level of pain and my inability to walk, I finally underwent back surgery.

Post-Surgical Reality and a Divine Turning Point

In 2015, I received a microdiscectomy procedure on my lower spine at the L4-S1 vertebrae. The surgery successfully removed the pressure on the compressed nerve root and thankfully restored my ability to walk. However, I was informed that the underlying spinal stenosis remained, along with permanent nerve damage due to the prolonged compression time. Not long after the surgery, the pain did not disappear; it simply shifted, appearing in various parts of my back above and below the surgical site, as well as in my ribs and rib cage. My upper back pain became more acute, and my legs would spontaneously give out. This physical crisis forced me to leave my job and begin exploring alternative ways to earn a living. I fell into a deep depression, feeling hopeless about my future.

Years before this, I had a profound religious experience that cemented my connection to God, a connection I rely on daily. However, during this time of post-surgical despair and hopelessness, I had a second, life-changing encounter. Lying in recovery, overwhelmed by my condition, I felt that my life was effectively over. In that moment, I turned to God in desperate prayer. The powerful, healing inspiration that followed did not just provide comfort; it guided me with precise clarity to begin the arduous, experimental journey of discovering a new path to wellness. This book, and the knowledge of the Roberts Method and the ABRM within it, is the culmination of that journey—a transformation from pain to healing, and from darkness to light. It is my deepest hope that this discovery will help countless others find relief from chronic pain.

Fun Fact: The pain you feel when you stub your toe actually travels from your toe to your brain at up to 200 miles per hour along specialized nerve fibers! However, the sharp, immediate pain travels on faster fibers than the dull, aching pain that follows.

PHOTO TAKEN IN 2015 AFTER BACK SURGERY (BEFORE METHOD USE)

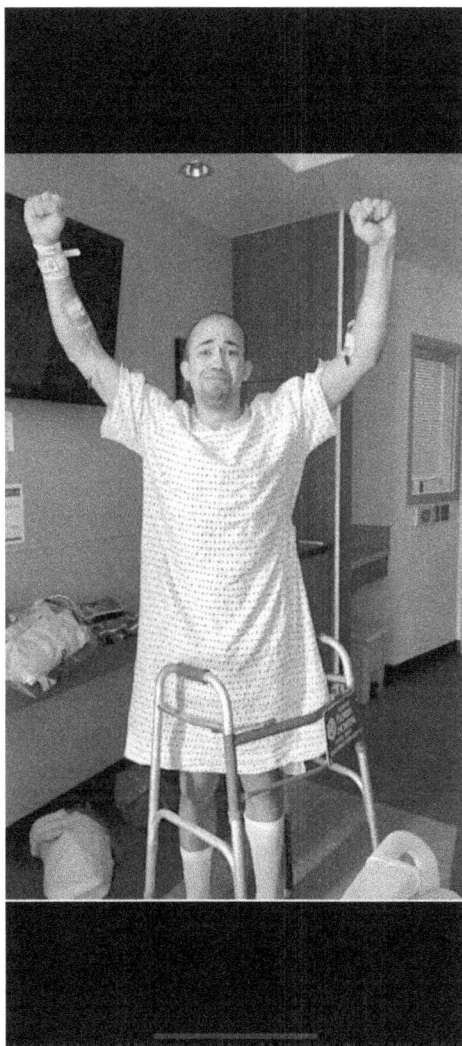

10 YEARS LATER. I STILL HAVE ARTHRITIS AND SPINAL STENOSIS.

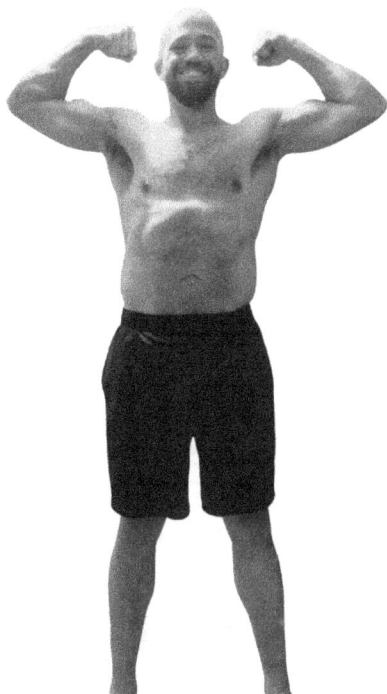

THE ELECTRICAL BLUEPRINT: PAIN, POSTURE, AND THE AUTONOMIC NERVOUS SYSTEM

T he profound intelligence that governs the human body oper-
ates far beneath the level of conscious awareness. Every complex
function—from the slightest movement and sensation to the body's
posture and emotional responses—is underpinned by an intricate
network of electrical communication. This vital signaling constantly
passes through the Central Nervous System (CNS), the Autonomic
Nervous System (ANS), and the sensory pathways deeply embedded
throughout our joints and connective tissues. Consequently, the experiences of pain, chronic tension, systemic imbalance, and the body's
self-healing responses are all direct expressions of these electrical systems at work, making every physical state a reflection of the nervous
system's current electrical map.

Understanding the Autonomic Nervous System (ANS) is paramount to grasping the mechanism of the ABR (Autonomic Bio Recovery) Maneuvers. The ANS functions as the body's hidden, automatic command center, diligently regulating essential involuntary
processes. Without any need for conscious input, it adjusts heart rate,
breathing, circulation, digestion, inflammation levels, body temper-
ature, and, critically, general muscle tone and posture. This system's
apparent invisibility is deceptive, as it maintains a direct connection to
conscious awareness through sensory perception. For instance, every
pain signal received and every subtle shift in tension noticed is a con-
sequence of the ANS delivering vital electrical information directly to
the brain, translating an autonomic event into a conscious experience.
The ABR Maneuvers are designed to interact directly with this system
by sending new, focused electrical signals. When a painful or restricted
area is stimulated, it triggers impulses that travel along the nerves,
into the spinal cord, and up to the brain. These signals function
as instructions, which the ANS interprets, leading it to predictably
modify the body's compensatory behavior. This inherent neurolog-

ical mechanism explains why pain often migrates through the body in recognizable patterns and why sustained relief can be achieved by following a specific, predictable sequence.

A lesser-known yet crucial role of the Autonomic Nervous System involves its profound control over posture and muscle behavior, particularly following an injury. In the immediate aftermath of tissue damage, the ANS reflexively alters tension patterns to instantly protect the compromised area. Muscles tighten, weight is involuntarily shifted to different joints, and the entire body adopts a guarded, compensatory posture—all before the injury is consciously registered. This protective reorganization by the ANS explains why chronic pain and tension often become established in areas far removed from the original site of injury; the body sacrifices overall mechanical balance to reduce strain on the injured spot. If the original injury is not fully resolved, this compensation is cemented, becoming the individual's "new normal" movement pattern. The ABR Maneuvers intervene in this chronic cycle by sending restorative electrical signals directly into the ANS, encouraging it to recalibrate and restore more natural, balanced movement patterns. Although the ANS is involuntary, it communicates constantly with consciousness through the mechanism of **interoception**—the awareness of internal sensations such as tension, heartbeat, breathing, and visceral pressure. When the ABR Maneuvers are applied, the user combines conscious attention with focused sensory stimulation, effectively giving the ANS a stream of new, corrective data to update its internal body map and guide a more accurate systemic response.

At its deepest level, pain is purely electrical. All sensory input—pain, pressure, warmth, numbness, and tingling—begins as electrical impulses generated by nerve endings. When tissue is irritated, specialized receptors called **nociceptors** fire electrical signals into the peripheral nerves, which carry the message toward the spinal cord and then ascend to the brain, where they are finally interpreted as the perception of pain. The entire process, from the nerve firing and signal transmission to the spinal cord's processing, the brain's interpretation, and the resulting motor and autonomic reflexes, is fundamentally electrical. Even emotional states like fear or stress alter pain perception by changing the electrical sensitivity of neurons. Furthermore, the **Articular Nervous System**, consisting of nerves embedded within joints, ligaments, capsules, and tendons, provides essential feedback about pressure, load, and position. This system is crucial, as it detects positional shifts, changes in weight distribution, and instability, serving to map and guide the physical **"movement of pain"** through the body's kinetic chain. When a painful area is relieved using the ABR Maneuvers, the articular nerves in the *next* joint in the sequence detect the suddenly increased load or stress, sending a signal that manifests as the migrating pain. This action, known as **Pain Migration**, reveals the body's predictable, nerve-guided sequence of compensation and release, a sequence the ABR Maneuvers simply allow the body to work through consciously and effectively. The ABR method integrates the CNS (for interpretation), the ANS (for automatic response), and the Articular Nervous System (for mechanical guidance), making it a comprehensive model for full-body recalibration.

Fun Fact: The **sympathetic** branch of the Autonomic Nervous System, which triggers the "fight or flight" response, can cause you to break out in goosebumps! This is a vestigial reflex from our distant ancestors, where making their hair stand up would have made them look larger and more threatening to a predator.

CHAPTER FIVE

THE CENTRAL COMMAND CENTER: WHY BACK PAIN IS BRAIN PAIN

I s your chronic back pain actually making it harder to think clearly? This chapter dives into the profound neurological reality: back injuries are not localized; they are systemic events that directly impact the entire central nervous system (CNS) and brain function. My own years-long battle with back pain—stemming from a herniated disc in my upper and lower spine, complicated by years of nerve compression leading to spinal stenosis—demonstrates this connection perfectly. By using the Roberts Method and Autonomic Bio Recovery (ABR)

Maneuvers, I was able to remove pain from both surface-level and deep-tissue injuries, transitioning from post-surgery agony to long periods of complete pain freedom. This lack of pain was not merely comfortable; it was the essential step that unlocked the ability to increase my flexibility, strength, and range of motion, and reclaim my cognitive function.

To understand why a severe back injury can affect your mood, memory, and personality, you must recognize the relationship between the brain and the spinal cord. They form the Central Nervous System (CNS), the body's primary control hub. The spinal cord is literally an extension of the brain, running down the back and protected by the vertebral column (the stacked vertebrae), which are cushioned by intervertebral discs. Layers of surrounding muscle also play a vital role in maintaining posture and protecting the spine. The spinal cord is a dense bundle of nerves that relays all signals between the brain and the body. Any injury to this column—whether a muscle strain, a herniated disc, or a direct spinal cord injury—can disrupt the flow of these signals, leading to profound neurological and psychological symptoms, including anxiety, depression, hopelessness, memory issues, and personality changes. Severe spine surgery is often considered a neurosurgical procedure because of this intimate connection.

When discussing how back injuries affect the brain, the key concept is Neuroplasticity—the brain's ability to reorganize itself. Unfortunately, chronic pain is a powerful driver of *negative* neuroplastic change. Persistent, unrelenting pain from nerve compression essentially highjacks the brain's control centers. Chronic pain physically alters the brain's pain-processing regions (like the somatosensory cortex), directly impacting cognitive functions such as attention, memory, and emotional regulation. This chronic signal overload has been linked to a measurable reduction in gray matter volume in areas of the brain associated with emotional and cognitive processing. Patients commonly report debilitating brain fog—difficulty concentrating and recalling information—because the brain is constantly preoccupied with processing the high-priority pain signals, leading to psychological conditions such as depression and anxiety.

Given the intricate relationship between back health and brain function, treatment must be holistic. The Autonomic Bio Recovery Maneuver (ABRM) is pivotal in this holistic approach. By systematically alleviating chronic muscle tension and gently improving spinal alignment, the ABRM can significantly reduce nerve strain and help restore proper, unimpeded signaling pathways between the spinal cord and the brain. Effective management is key to reversing the cognitive and emotional impacts. Encouraging physical activity, improving posture, and strengthening core muscles are essential components of a recovery plan. The ABRM's role is to remove the pain that *prevents* you from safely exercising and maintaining a healthy posture. By addressing back injuries with this comprehensive approach—early intervention, targeted self-care techniques like ABRM, and holistic rehabilitation—it is possible not only to alleviate pain but to improve overall brain function, memory, and emotional well-being.

Fun Fact: The Vagus Nerve, the longest cranial nerve, runs from the brainstem to the abdomen and is heavily influenced by spinal alignment and chronic tension. It plays a key role in regulating mood, anxiety, and inflammation, demonstrating a direct, physical pathway between your spine's health and your mental state.

CHAPTER SIX

THE HIDDEN COST OF COMPENSATION & WHY YOUR BODY LIES TO YOU

Have you ever injured your ankle only to develop knee or hip pain months later? This seemingly unrelated discomfort is the handiwork of **muscle compensation**, a natural, instinctive, and often subconscious response where one part of the body sacrifices its own health to shield a weakened or injured area. When trauma occurs—be it a sprained ligament, a torn muscle, or a severe sprain—your body automatically adapts to avoid immediate pain, allowing you to maintain a semblance of normal functioning. However, this protective mechanism comes with significant negative side effects. Understanding what drives and sustains muscle compensation is not just useful, but **crucial** for effective pain management, successful rehabilitation, and achieving optimal, long-term physical function.

The Anatomy of Avoidance: Conscious vs. Subconscious Shifts

When an injury occurs, mobility is immediately limited, and the natural reaction is to minimize the use of the damaged area. If you injure a hand, you rely more heavily on the other; if you sprain a knee, you shift your body weight onto the unaffected leg to minimize load. This phenomenon is deeply embedded in our biology, similar to how a person who loses their sight often develops a heightened sense of hearing. The root cause of compensation is simple: the inherent drive to avoid pain. This compensatory action can be **conscious** (like intentionally favoring one leg), but it is often **subconscious**, manifesting as a subtle, constant alteration of posture or movement patterns.

Compensation is not confined to large, visible muscle groups; it infiltrates smaller stabilizing muscles and the complex web of connective tissues. When one muscle group is forced into overuse to protect an injured or weakened spot, it triggers a cascade of biomechanical changes throughout the body. Muscles, tendons, ligaments, and even joints are forced to operate in ways they are **not anatomically designed to handle**. This results in additional, *secondary* pain, uneven weight distribution, muscular effort imbalance, and progressive misalignment of the body's natural posture. This altered, maladaptive posture can trigger a chain reaction, affecting everything from overall spinal alignment to the long-term health of distant joints.

The Central Role of the Spine and Brain

The integrity of the spine is central to this discussion, as it is wrapped in layers of interconnected muscles and connective tissue that span the entire body. If you compensate for an injury, you inevitably overuse or underuse specific spinal muscles, leading to imbalance. Lack of muscle use leads to **muscle atrophy** (weakening). When the stabilizing muscles surrounding the spine weaken, the full extent of the structural damage, both present and ongoing, becomes impossible to accurately assess. The discs in the spine function much like a precisely stacked assembly line, with each vertebra receiving specific instructions from the brain stem. If an injury slows or cuts off these lines of communication, the negative side effects can ripple far beyond the mechanical: communication disruptions in the brain stem can lead to memory deficits, cognitive impairments, headaches, mood swings, anxiety, and depression. Fortunately, the **brain compensates** as well, exhibiting an amazing ability known as **neuroplasticity**—rewiring itself and forming new neural connections to reroute information.

However, the spinal structure remains vulnerable. If you injure one small part of a disc, the impact is structural and systemic. Think of the spine as a stack of bricks: a seemingly minor hairline crack in one brick can compromise the strength and integrity of the entire column. If that compromise is near the base, the shift and change in the entire structure are easily observed. Because compensation and weight distribution are fundamental laws of physics, the **Autonomic Bio Recovery Maneuvers (ABRM)** must address these principles directly. To effectively treat a damaged or weakened spinal area, you must not only stimulate the pain point but also stimulate the exact **opposite part of the vertebrae** to which the pain is connected. Furthermore, you must systematically stimulate every muscle and connective tissue in all directions from the original injury to ensure complete pain removal.

The Consequences of Prolonged Compensation

While muscle compensation is initially a protective mechanism, its prolonged use accelerates wear and tear, leading to significant, negative, and long-term implications. For example, over-relying on one leg due to a knee injury places undue stress on the hip, knee, or ankle joints of the *unaffected* side, leading to accelerated degeneration and potentially **osteoarthritis**. This uneven pressure on the musculoskeletal structure creates what I term **secondary pain points**. These muscle imbalances cause specific muscles to become overactive and tight while others become weak and inhibited. An individual compensating for a hip issue by favoring the opposite leg might subsequently develop back pain, secondary knee issues, or even **plantar fasciitis** due to the resulting altered gait and biomechanics.

Crucially, compensation can effectively mask the original injury by generating overwhelming secondary pain, often delaying proper diagnosis and prolonging recovery. This phenomenon, known as **pain migration**, occurs because the brain tends to focus on the most intense or most recent pain signal rather than its true source. When you want to remove the pain using the Roberts Method, you must strategically address and remove these **newer compensation pains first**, before the older, primary injury can be properly addressed and removed. Over time, the body's new, compromised posture can become the **maladaptive postural pattern**, effectively resetting the body's neutral alignment, making a return to true balance impossible without deliberate, targeted intervention.

The Path to Balance with the Roberts Method

Addressing muscle compensation is essential for complete recovery and preventing future complications. Simply relieving pain in one area without accounting for the compensatory changes throughout the entire body will inevitably set the stage for new problems to arise.

The **Roberts Method** and the **Autonomic Bio Recovery Maneuvers** teach you how to **"navigate through your pain path,"** which involves systematically finding and addressing every single primary and secondary point of pain and dysfunction. This process requires patience and a thorough understanding of the body's interconnected systems.

The goal is to reverse these maladaptive patterns and gradually return the body to its natural neutral position, where muscles, joints, and connective tissues function optimally without undue strain. This holistic approach involves not just the ABRM, but also a commitment to complementary practices like **weight training**, targeted **exercise**, **flexibility training**, **stretching**, and regular activity. By ending pain and restoring function to the injured parts, you eliminate the **need** for compensation. The subsequent focus shifts to rebalancing the musculoskeletal system: strengthening underactive muscles and releasing tension in overactive ones. This enhances overall mobility, stability, and coordination, which is critical for preventing falls, improving performance, and maintaining a high quality of life. The longer and greater the compensation has been, the more focused rehabilitation will be required. By navigating your pain path, you can uncover hidden sources of discomfort, restore your body's natural alignment, and promote long-term health and vitality.

Fun Fact: The **fascia**, the thin casing of connective tissue surrounding muscles and organs, acts like a full-body "spiderweb." Because it is continuous, tension from an old injury in your big toe can literally pull on the tissue all the way up your leg and into your shoulder, explaining why compensation patterns are rarely localized!

CHAPTER SEVEN

THE ILLUSION OF MOVEMENT & WHY PAIN ONLY SEEMS TO TRAVEL

Have you ever felt a deep, dull ache disappear from your lower back, only to have a sharp pain instantly flare up in your opposite hip or shoulder? This isn't pain physically "moving" through your body; it's an **illusion of migration** created by your nervous system's shifting focus. This phenomenon is governed by **Sensory Dominance**: the principle that the most intense electrical signal—the loudest alarm—always commands the brain's full attention. When you successfully use the **Autonomic Bio Recovery Maneu-**

vers **(ABRM)** to silence that primary, dominant pain, your mind immediately shifts awareness to the **next loudest signal**—a secondary muscle group that was already quietly hurting but was previously masked by the intense primary pain. In this chapter, we will examine the sensations experienced as pain progresses during healing, investigate how pain seems to hide beneath numbness, and learn how to methodically reveal and resolve it.

The Hierarchical Nature of Pain: Tertiary Points and Hiding Sensations

Pain, at its core, has a source point, but injuries can, and usually do, create multiple, stacked sources. In earlier chapters, we discussed primary and secondary pain points; after successfully addressing those, seemingly **"new" pain** may emerge in other areas, which I refer to as **tertiary pain points**. This process of pain *emerging* is a physiological unpacking that can take differing amounts of time. Deeper pains can reveal themselves immediately after removing a main pain point, or they can take months or even years to surface. These "hidden" pains are often masked by **numbness** or a low-grade, constant discomfort that the brain learned to filter out long ago, treating it as background noise. The process of combining the ABR Maneuvers with a holistic rehabilitation approach gives you the power to consciously override this filtering system and restore your body.

A critical concept for tracking these deeper pains is **Upward Stacking**. Pain and tension have a natural tendency to stack hierarchically. Think of it like a ripple effect: the pain radiates outward in waves that you can feel, track, and mark as you recover. However, it's not just horizontal; the cumulative effect of tension from the feet, knees, and hips stacks pressure upwards into the spine and head, contributing to the complexity of treatment. Because the body will store muscle tension without a natural process that reliably releases it, you must actively intervene to lessen and remove it using the Roberts Method.

Facial Tension and the Deep Reservoirs of Stress

Stored muscle tension serves as an excellent marker for locating deep, hard-to-find pains throughout the entire body. **Muscle tension** signifies a muscle that is involuntarily tense or flexed at a resting point. If this tension is persistent enough, it transitions from simple tightness into genuine pain. This tension exists all over the body, including the face and head, where it is both surface-level and **deeply rooted**. Over time, this deep facial tension can contribute to the formation of hard lines and wrinkles. The face and head are wrapped in numerous layers of muscle; persistent tension here is why headaches often occur, signaling a stress overload in these neurological reservoirs.

By consciously engaging the ABR Maneuvers, you can help lessen and release this stored tension and these **trigger points**, not just in the face and head, but across the body's entire musculature. Undoing this stored muscle tension and dissolving deep compensatory patterns is often a labor-intensive, lengthy task, but the journey is its own reward. The road to recovery is paved with countless small and large victories.

Restoring Function and Reversing Atrophy

After successfully removing a significant pain point, you begin to use a muscle, limb, or group of muscles that may have been intentionally avoided for years. As you restore function to previously injured areas, you naturally reveal additional and deeper compensation patterns. In my own recovery, it has taken years to reverse the chronic damage in my spine and manage full-body pain. After the initial fall at age fourteen, the muscles in my back that I instinctively disengaged lost strength and began to **atrophy** (waste away). The prolonged effects of arthritis and spinal stenosis led to significant muscle wasting and disc height loss. While arthritis is incurable, I can consistently manage the pain using the ABR Maneuvers. Despite the risk of pain returning due to stress or re-injury, I lead an active life, enjoying running, swimming, basketball, and participating in sports with my children—a life that was unimaginable when I was unable to walk.

In 2015, I was completely unable to walk or stand due to the cumulative strain of years of muscle compensation and atrophy. My body had spent years compensating for pain by avoiding certain movements, and eventually, the system collapsed. However, this cycle of degeneration **can be broken**. Using the Roberts Method, I was able to reverse the damage, restore strength, and increase vitality. While the self-diagnosis and development process took me seven years, you now have a guide with all my experience, making your journey much quicker.

The Art of Navigating the Pain Path

The human body is complex, and pain can be elusive. The process of systematically finding deeply hidden pain to achieve true, lasting relief is what I call **"navigating through your pain path."** This journey requires dedication, but the rewards are profound: regaining control over your body, ending chronic pain, and returning to a life of activity and vitality.

Throughout this process, you will learn to truly listen to your body and understand its signals. Pain is not merely a nuisance to be suppressed; it is critical information signaling that a problem needs to be addressed. By paying attention to these signals and using the ABR Method, you can restore your body's natural, balanced state. This method is not about short-term fixes; it is about restoring the body's natural balance and preventing future injuries. By identifying the *source* of the pain and addressing its **upward stacking** and **outward radiating waves** directly, you can achieve long-term control. The Roberts Method is a complex phenomenon made manageable, a process that is achievable by anyone willing to commit the time and dedication.

Fun Fact: **Referred pain**, like the famous phenomenon where heart trouble causes pain in the left arm, is a type of sensory confusion where the brain misinterprets the origin of a signal. This happens because the visceral nerves (from the organs) and the somatic nerves (from the skin and muscles) converge on the same neurons in the spinal cord, causing the brain to incorrectly "map" the painful sensation.

CHAPTER EIGHT

THE UNAVOIDABLE SLIDE: CAN WE REALLY FIGHT AGE-RELATED BREAKDOWN?

A s the human body journeys through the decades, maintaining muscle strength, tone, volume, and overall structural integrity becomes an increasing challenge. Muscles that were once firm begin to lose their tone, exhibiting what appears to be a natural sag. Joints endure wear and tear from years of cumulative use, and tendons lose their thickness and stability, making them significantly more prone to injury. This inevitable process is often referred to as aging, but the real enemy is **"age-related breakdown"**—a systemic decline that diminishes vitality. The critical question isn't whether we can *reverse* aging, but whether we can effectively **slow down its debilitating effects**, extending the period of life where one remains active, vibrant, and fully functional. The fight begins with understanding the smallest enemy: **micro-degradation**.

The Silent Saboteur: Micro-Degradation

To truly confront physical decline, we must first understand **micro-degradation**. This concept explains the small, often unnoticeable, yet continuous loss of minute muscle fibers or muscle tension that can occur anywhere, both internally and externally. Micro-degradation of muscle tissue can be defined as the gradual, microscopic breakdown of muscle fibers and tissues primarily due to inactivity or insufficient use. Muscles that are not regularly engaged in physical activity rapidly begin to lose size, strength, and endurance. Over time, this subtle process spreads and compounds, resulting in widespread negative effects, including reduced overall function and a heightened susceptibility to major injuries. This challenge is acutely personal: in my full-time career, spending forty hours a week sitting and standing behind a desk exacerbates my prior back injuries. If I remain seated for too long, I feel a painful sense of spinal compression, leading to localized lower back pain and noticeable weakness in my legs.

Micro-degradation compounds problems dramatically for those with already **inactive lifestyles** and, critically, for those with **injured muscles**. When muscle tissue is damaged, the body instinctively protects it by compensating, leading to non-use of the injured part. This compensation accelerates atrophy and deterioration in the weakened area. The breakdown of muscle tissue due to micro-degradation can cause a wide range of issues, including numbness in the extremities, functional loss, cognitive decline (like brain fog), sexual dysfunction, and a pervasive decrease in overall quality of life. This process is subtle yet pervasive, often beginning much earlier than most people realize—even sedentary young adults or teenagers can experience its onset, as muscle strength and flexibility require constant, regular stimulation. Without it, the microscopic breakdown accelerates.

The Age Factor and The ABR Countermeasure

For many individuals, micro-degradation begins in their **mid-twenties**, a period when the body's natural production of growth hormones and other **anabolic processes** (which support muscle repair and growth) naturally starts its slow decline. As a result, muscles that aren't actively used lose their ability to regenerate efficiently. This process accelerates for older adults, leading to more pronounced muscle loss and weakness, a condition clinically known as **sarcopenia**.

The **Autonomic Bio Recovery Maneuvers (ABRM)** offer a promising, direct approach to counteracting this muscle decline and managing associated pain. By systematically working through and stimulating each muscle group, the technique helps to **reawaken and retrain** muscles that have been dormant, lost coordination, or have atrophied due to compensation. As these inhibited muscles regain their functional vitality, **muscle memory**—often thought to be lost—can return rapidly. This physical rejuvenation achieved through neurological stimulation often translates directly into **mental rejuvenation**, helping to mitigate the cognitive toll of chronic pain.

Strategies for Graceful Aging

While the fight against aging is one we cannot entirely win, we can equip ourselves with effective methods to navigate it more gracefully. Aging naturally involves muscle breakdown, but regular exercise and a balanced diet are proven to mitigate many adverse effects. Research indicates that maintaining a positive, active, and healthy lifestyle enhances the production of essential hormones, including dopamine, serotonin, and melatonin, which are crucial for regulating mood, energy, and overall well-being.

However, lifestyle adjustments alone are often insufficient. Many people exercise regularly and eat well yet still face the inevitable decline. The **Roberts Method** is one such strategy that supports graceful aging by addressing muscle soreness and promoting continuous activity. When muscle soreness and pain are significantly reduced or removed, the body is naturally less inclined to become sedentary, which is the primary accelerator of physical decline. Staying active is essential for maintaining muscle strength, flexibility, and overall vitality, as regular movement encourages blood flow, delivers vital nutrients, and prevents the accumulation of waste products like lactic acid that contribute to stiffness.

The Science of Decline and Recovery

Understanding the science behind muscle aging reveals that the decline is caused by a decrease in the number and size of muscle fibers, a reduction in proteins needed for repair, and the deterioration of **motor neurons** that control muscle contraction. Emerging research shows that **resistance training and weight-bearing exercises** are key to stimulating muscle protein synthesis, helping to maintain mass and strength. Additionally, specific dietary interventions, such as increased protein intake and supplements like creatine, can support muscle preservation. By integrating the **Self-Adjustment Technique** (ABRM) to address the underlying neurological and compensation issues with regular exercise, proper nutrition, and mental engagement, one can establish a robust framework for aging. The goal is not just to live longer, but to live *better*, maintaining the highest possible physical and mental function throughout life.

Fun Fact: When astronauts return from space, they can lose up to **20% of their muscle mass** in a matter of weeks, primarily because the lack of gravity prevents muscles from receiving the necessary **weight-bearing stimulus** required to fight off micro-degradation. This rapid effect highlights how crucial consistent external load is for maintaining muscle integrity.

CHAPTER NINE

STEP 1: FINDING PAIN POINTS AND THE THREE-POINT STIMULATION TECHNIQUE

Have you ever pressed on a sore spot, only to find the real pain was radiating deeper or shifting to an adjacent area? That sensation reveals the core truth of pain: it is never truly isolated.

This chapter introduces the crucial first stage of the Roberts Method: Step 1: Finding Pain Points, and the innovative technique required to address them effectively, the Three-Point Stimulation Technique (3PST). No matter where or how many places you feel pain, this methodical search and comprehensive stimulation will always be the starting point. As covered in earlier chapters, the foundational concepts of ABR Maneuvers allow you to predict pain migration; here, we put that knowledge into action.

The primary objective of Step 1 is simple: Find the most painful area of your body. You can approach this systematically by addressing one chronic point at a time, or, preferably, by assessing multiple regions of discomfort simultaneously. A helpful guideline is that the more points you target at once, the more strength you will regain and the more significant the reduction in pain you will experience due to the comprehensive neurological reset. Once you locate a specific muscle or joint point, effective stimulation is crucial. Start by applying gentle pressure, then gradually increase the intensity as needed and as tolerated. The reason for this gradual but increasing intensity is that deeper pressure is necessary to reach the underlying layers of tissue where the root of chronic pain often originates. Visualize a significant impact creating a crater in a foam mattress; the deepest damage lies beneath the surface bruise. Identifying all core impact or damage points from your original injury—not just the surface pain—is vital to achieving a complete recovery.

I discovered the need for the 3PST while treating severe, resistant arthritis pain in my upper spine. Stimulating a single point in isolation proved insufficient for injuries involving deep, complex structures like vertebral discs or joints with numerous tendon attachments. The Three-Point Stimulation Technique (3PST) addresses pain in these complex, hard-to-reach areas by simultaneously targeting a minimum of three interconnected points within the affected region. This technique forms the foundation of the Roberts Method for complex pain, accelerating recovery by addressing the interconnected structures that contribute to pain. The first rule of my method is clear: If you cannot stimulate the areas where you are in pain, you cannot remove that pain. For spinal pain, you would use a firm surface (like the corner of a wall) to apply pressure to the main, most sensitive pain point on the affected vertebra, while simultaneously stimulating the muscles or vertebrae immediately superior (above) and immediately inferior (below) to it. You would also use your hands to find additional sensitive points in the ribs or supporting muscles adjacent to the spine while applying the main pressure. Stimulating three or more points simultaneously ensures the pressure reaches not only the primary pain source but also the necessary stabilizing structures that have gone into chronic compensatory spasm.

The 3PST is equally effective for joint pain, such as in the knees, which are complex systems where ligaments, tendons, and surrounding muscles work together to maintain dynamic balance. To treat a joint effectively, you must identify the primary area of tenderness and then target the muscle/tendon attachment points proximal (above) and distal (below) the joint. This technique aligns with scientific principles of structural interdependence and neurological gate control. The Gate Control Theory of Pain suggests that non-painful input (like the firm pressure applied by 3PST) can effectively "close the gates" to painful input, preventing the pain signals from reaching the brain. By stimulating multiple points, you flood the sensory pathways with corrective input, overwhelming and temporarily closing the pain gate. This methodical approach may initially feel like a "pain journey" as you uncover deeply rooted discomfort, but as you progress, it transforms into a true "healing journey," building resilience and vitality.

Fun Fact: The Gate Control Theory of Pain suggests that non-painful input (like the firm pressure applied by 3PST) can effectively "close the gates" to painful input, preventing the pain signals from reaching the brain. By stimulating three points at once, you flood the sensory pathways with corrective input, overwhelming and temporarily closing the pain gate.

CHAPTER TEN

THE MECHANICS OF RECALIBRATION: STEPS 2 THROUGH 5 OF THE ABR MANEUVERS

The core of the Autonomic Bio Recovery Method (ABRM) lies in using controlled movements and targeted pressure to generate specific sensory input, encouraging the nervous system to recalibrate compensatory tension patterns. This chapter details the final four mechanical steps that follow the foundational "Finding Pain Points" (Step 1), designed to systematically release tension from the extremities and spine.

Step 2: Arm Flexion and Synovial Release

Following the deep compression of the targeted pain points from Step 1, Step 2 focuses on neurological release in the upper extremity. While maintaining firm pressure on the painful area identified in Step 1, bend your left arm toward your body and flex the muscle forcefully. Next, while still maintaining the deep compression, straighten your arm vigorously. If executed correctly, you may hear a distinct "pop" in your left elbow. This sound is not indicative of structural damage; rather, it is the result of rapid movement of synovial fluid and gases within the joint capsule, which is the mechanism of temporary joint release and is considered a desirable sign of progress. It is important to note that this step may not work for every individual. Some may struggle to apply sufficient pressure or generate a forceful enough flex and extension to elicit the pop. If you are unable to complete this step, simply proceed directly to Step 3, as the overall effectiveness of the subsequent steps will not be compromised.

Step 3: Head and Neck (Atlas & Axis) Rotation

Once Step 2 is complete, you will move to releasing tension in the cervical spine. Ensure you are in a comfortable standing or lying down position. Begin by purposefully scrunching your shoulders towards your neck while simultaneously applying substantial downward pressure on your head (either with your hands or by carefully pressing your head against a wall/firm surface). Hold still in this position of maximum compression and tension, and then slowly rotate your head clockwise. During this rotation, listen carefully for popping or clicking sounds; these audible releases are normal and are desirable signs that tension is being released from the deep structures of the neck, including the Atlas and Axis vertebrae (C1 and C2). If you do not hear any sounds despite completing the previous steps, it may signify that insufficient pressure was applied in Step 1. In this case, you should return to Step 1 and apply more pressure to the affected areas before returning to and proceeding with the subsequent steps.

Step 4: Lower Body Connection and Deep Squat Release

Step 4 systematically introduces the lower body into the recalibration sequence. Start by standing upright, then slowly and intentionally squat down to your ankles, allowing your body to briefly rest in this maximally flexed position. The goal is to maximize the pressure within the knee and ankle joints, which should elicit a noticeable popping sensation from your knees and/or ankles. If you do not hear any sounds upon reaching this position, repeat the step by gently bouncing on your ankles to generate the necessary release. Afterward, smoothly rise back up to standing, first elevating onto your tiptoes (full plantar flexion) and then slowly returning to a flat stance. This full range of motion primes the lower body joints. If you have followed these steps correctly, the neurological connection between your upper and lower body should be optimized for the final, targeted release.

Step 5: The Right Knee Turn (Final Integration)

Step 5 is the final, targeted maneuver and should be performed with caution to prevent injury. After completing Step 4 and standing straight, shift all your body weight onto your right foot, simultaneously lifting your left leg off the ground. While keeping your right foot firmly planted and stable, gently and slowly turn your entire body and the lifted left leg to the left (counterclockwise). The goal of this rotation is to create a shearing or releasing force in the stabilizing structures of the weighted knee. You should hear and feel a significant pop in your inner knee joint. If this targeted joint release occurs, you have successfully completed the full sequence of the Autonomic Bio Recovery Technique. By following these steps sequentially, you are now equipped with the practical knowledge to perform the Roberts Method and its accompanying ABRM maneuvers effectively, empowering you on your journey toward recovery and wellness.

Fun Fact: The popping sound heard in joints is known scientifically as tribonucleation. It occurs when a sudden distraction of the joint space creates a vacuum bubble that rapidly collapses, releasing the gases (primarily carbon dioxide) dissolved in the synovial fluid. The action of the ABRM uses this physical mechanism to create a powerful sensory input for the brain.

Chapter Eleven

TIPS TO USE THE ABR MANEUVERS MORE EFFECTIVELY. REMOVING COMPLEX AND DEEP MUSCLE PAIN. HOW TO USE

POSITIONING AND WEIGHTS TO TARGET AND REMOVE DEEP PAIN AND HARD-TO-REACH MUSCLES PAIN; AS WELL

AS JOINT RELATED PAIN.

The Roberts Method and ABR Maneuvers should be used on a muscle or disc in three separate states — inactive, compressed, and flexed — to alleviate pain resulting from an injury effectively. Each state targets various aspects of muscle tension and pain pathways, ensuring comprehensive relief and promoting recovery.

1. The Inactive or Neutral Position

The first foundational position for clicking it out involves addressing the muscle when it is inactive. An inactive muscle is one that is not moving and is not under any external force or pressure. In this state, the muscle is relaxed, allowing for a more precise identification of pain points and their underlying causes. By focusing on the inactive muscle, you can release tension and identify latent pain that may not be apparent during movement. It is critical to perform techniques, such as gentle massage or manipulation, on the relaxed muscle without applying any force. This allows the muscle fibers to release tension and recalibrate gradually without further strain.

2. Combing the ABR Maneuvers with Direct Compression

The second technique involves manually applying pressure to the muscle around the pain through compression, squeezing, or using a blunt object to stimulate the affected area. This approach directly engages the muscle fibers, fascia, and associated tissues where pain is present, easing the breakdown of adhesions and releasing muscle knots. By applying targeted pressure, you can increase blood flow to the area and accelerate the removal of metabolic waste products contributing to pain and inflammation.

In this position, the muscle stays inactive but is subjected to intentional compression. The application of pressure helps identify specific pain points that may otherwise go unnoticed and offers an opportunity for more effective adjustments. It is essential to use the ABR Maneuvers in this state carefully to prevent any adding stored tension, strain, or injury.

3. Apply the ABR Maneuvers while attempting to flex the muscle of the injury.

The third critical position involves using the ABR Maneuvers while the muscle is flexed. In this state, the muscle is contracted. Targeting muscle pain while the muscle is flexed can help reveal hidden pain points that are only noticeable under certain conditions. To achieve this, apply resistance by pushing or pulling against an object, such as a wall, or using tools to prod and stimulate the pain. This step is crucial for identifying pain that may not be apparent when the muscle relaxes.

The next step in this process is the most vital. In addition to applying pressure and flexing the sore muscle or area, specific muscles may require you to use this technique in multiple positions. It is essential to search for pain actively; if you do not, you may not achieve complete pain relief. For example, body parts such as joints and vertebrae must be adaptable to the constant shifts in weight and pressure they endure daily. In addition to stretching, you can also combine the ABR Maneuvers with the added use of weight or resistance. Resistances can add substantially more pressure to a painful area. This can help to stimulate deeper muscle tissue to be able to use the ABR Maneuvers most effectively. Therefore, to truly become pain-free, you should try various positions with weights or resistance bands to find all the areas where pain lives. This thorough exploration alleviates pain and offers several benefits, including increased strength, improved circulation, enhanced range of motion, and improved health.

It is essential to note that muscle or surrounding tissue pain sometimes appears to shift or relocate. This perception is often due to the brain's interpretation of pain signals based on their intensity rather than the actual location of the problem. Pain may exist in multiple areas simultaneously, but the brain prioritizes the most intense signal. Once the ABR Maneuvers have been applied to alleviate pain on a damaged area, you may experience subtle posture, balance, and overall musculoskeletal alignment shifts.

The autonomic bio recovery maneuvers are not only about addressing pain, they also involve a comprehensive understanding of how pain signals interact within the musculoskeletal system, autonomic nervous system, and the brain. This concept emphasizes the importance of thoroughly identifying and addressing all areas of pain, regardless of location. The phenomenon of perceived pain migration highlights the importance of examining all sources of discomfort within the affected muscle groups. This comprehensive approach is crucial for alleviating pain and promoting overall health.

Pain is a vital signal from the brain that shows an underlying issue that requires attention. Rather than merely being an obstacle to overcome, pain guides you to areas that need adjustment and healing. By understanding and following your pain path, you can identify and address the root causes of discomfort, paving the way for adequate recovery and triggering the body's natural healing processes.

CHAPTER TWELVE

THE GROUND-UP SOLUTION: WHY KNEE PAIN STARTS IN YOUR FEET

H ave you ever treated a leaky roof without checking the foundation? When it comes to chronic knee pain, focusing only on the joint is often the same mistake. While the knee may hurt, the true source of your discomfort—and the key to lasting relief—often lies far below, in your feet. This chapter shares my journey of overcoming persistent, chronic knee pain, revealing a crucial discovery about the body's intricate kinetic chain, and providing a systematic approach to applying the Autonomic Bio Recovery Method (ABRM) to find relief, starting from the ground up.

The Frustration of Surface-Level Treatment

Initially, recovering my knees with the ABRM was deeply frustrating. I focused strictly on the primary pain points within the joint itself, applying the method to the exact spot that hurt the most. While this provided temporary relief, the pain invariably returned. I knew the ABRM worked—I had used it successfully on my back and shoulders—but something about the knee was fundamentally different. I then expanded my focus, addressing multiple pain points *around* the knee, but still achieved only marginal, temporary improvement. Movements like climbing stairs or turning sharply continued to cause sharp pain, and I constantly lacked confidence in my ability to move freely. It felt as though my body was telling me that my efforts were structurally incomplete.

Then the key realization hit me: the knees are not isolated. They are a crucial shock-absorbing hinge within a much larger, interconnected kinetic system. Like the spine, the knees rely entirely on stable support from surrounding structures—muscles, tendons, ligaments, and bones—for stability and proper function. To achieve permanent knee pain relief, I had to look far beyond the joint and address the entire compensatory chain of connections, beginning with the feet.

The Foundation of the Body: Feet and Alignment

Your feet are quite literally the foundation of your body's posture and mechanics. Any imbalance, misalignment, or weakness in this foundation directly affects the position and stability of the knees, hips, and other joints further up the chain. When you walk, stand, or rest, the distribution of weight and pressure across your feet dictates the alignment of your entire leg. Uneven pressure, whether caused by inherited structure, worn-out shoes, or an old, unnoticed injury, instantly strains the tendons and muscles in your legs. For example, consistently placing more weight on the outer edge of one foot (supination) initiates a chain reaction: the ankle rolls outward, the knee collapses inward to compensate, the hip tilts, and the strain radiates up to create tension in your lower back. This explains why it is essential to address the root cause of knee pain by starting with the feet.

The ABRM provides a systematic, ground-up approach to identifying and alleviating pain in your feet, knees, and the entire compensatory structure. You start by using a tool, such as a firm ball, roller, or even a solid water bottle, to apply pressure to the soles of your feet. Initially, you gently step or stand on the tool, methodically moving your feet to find tender or painful areas. As you stimulate these points, you often uncover deeper layers of discomfort in the connected tissues. The more pressure you apply (within your pain tolerance), the deeper the tissue layer you address, allowing you to access and remove tension from deep fascia and musculature that has been chronically compensating for years. This process helps restore proper nerve function and reawaken dormant muscles and tendons from the ground up.

The Role of Nerves and Fascia in Pain Migration

The body is a marvel of interconnected systems. Misalignment in the feet creates stress that can travel upward, affecting the knees, hips, shoulders, and even the neck. This cascade of pain is explained by the intricate roles of nerves and fascia (the continuous web of connective tissue surrounding muscles and organs). The soles of your feet are incredibly rich in nerve endings that communicate with the entire body. Stimulating these nerves through the ABRM can help reduce pain perception and improve overall proprioception (awareness of where your body is in space). Additionally, tight or damaged fascia in the feet can hold chronic tension that travels the length of the leg, contributing to knee discomfort. By using the ABRM to release this fascia, you address hidden sources of discomfort and promote long-term stability.

Once pain is significantly reduced, the next step is crucial: rebuilding strength and stability. Incorporate simple movements like toe raises, gentle lunges, or balance exercises to retrain your muscles and reinforce proper alignment. This process ensures your body adapts to its new, pain-free position and prevents compensatory patterns from re-emerging. Healing does not end when the pain is gone; maintaining healthy knees and feet requires ongoing care, including supportive footwear, good posture, and daily self-massage. Your mindset also plays a crucial role; stress and tension are stored physically, and practicing mindfulness and patience enhances the effectiveness of the ABRM.

Fun Fact: Your feet contain 26 bones, 33 joints, and over 100 muscles, tendons, and ligaments, acting as complex spring systems. This intricate structure is the only part of your body that constantly absorbs forces equivalent to 1.5 times your body weight with every step you take, explaining why even a minor misalignment there can cause major joint distress

CHAPTER THIRTEEN

THE BODY'S WEAKEST LINK: HOW SHOULDER PAIN BECAME A ROADMAP TO HEALING

D id you know the complex pain in your shoulder could actually be limiting the strength in your fingers? While previous chapters touched on the systemic effects of trauma, particularly the atrophy caused by disuse, this chapter focuses intensely on the shoulder joint—the body's most mobile yet most vulnerable compound muscle group. My journey through chronic pain was constantly hampered by repeated shoulder injuries, which served as a relentless reminder of how interconnected, fragile, and resilient the human body truly is. I share here the challenging, labor-intensive recovery processes that followed each incident, which ultimately forced me to refine and prove the efficacy of the Autonomic Bio Recovery Maneuvers (ABRM).

The Origin of Instability: Spinal Connection

The genesis of my shoulder problems can be directly traced back to the initial trauma of falling down the stairs at age fourteen. This incident resulted in a herniated disc in my upper back (cervical/thoracic spine), which later developed into debilitating arthritis. During severe episodes related to the spinal injury, my ability to lift my arms was severely restricted. This forced disuse led directly to significant muscle weakness and atrophy in the associated shoulder and arm musculature. The chronic pain and loss of mobility were constant, clear signals demonstrating that a weakness in the spine—the body's electrical highway—had immediate, cascading effects on the kinetic chain linking the back, shoulder, and arm.

In addition to this spinal atrophy, I sustained numerous acute shoulder injuries that compounded the damage. These included improperly lifting a heavy object, which resulted in a separate, agonizing shoulder separation; two distinct instances of trauma related to seizures (once falling and breaking a power outlet, and another time falling out of bed directly onto the shoulder); and a separate strain sustained while attempting to dunk a basketball. I once loved sports, but the cumulative effect of these injuries eventually instilled a deep-seated fear of physical activity, hindering both my physical and emotional well-being for years.

The Challenge of Complexity: Anatomy and Compensation

Healing a complex muscle group like the shoulders requires a highly nuanced understanding of its interdependent anatomy. The shoulder is supported by approximately twenty distinct muscles, which are vital for the joint's movement, stability, and rotation. This interconnectedness means an injury to just one muscle—or an instability caused by spinal weakness—has a cascading, compensatory effect on all others. Crucially, shoulder pain rarely stops at the joint; it often radiates down the arms, affecting muscle control and, as mentioned, can even extend to negatively impact hand strength and finger dexterity.

A minor injury often escalates into a major chronic issue because it leads to compensatory movements that worsen the initial problem. For instance, constantly hiking the shoulder to avoid pain in the rotator cuff creates tension in the neck and spine, forming a cycle of dysfunction. The unique structure of the shoulder, with its high range of motion, limits its ability to heal independently from severe trauma, sometimes necessitating medical interventions like surgery. However, my technique offers an alternative pathway to functional recovery, allowing individuals to rebuild robust, pain-free shoulders.

The Painful Proof: Applying the ABRM

After discovering my self-healing method, I was eager to apply it to my severely damaged shoulders. Even after I successfully managed and ended my severe spinal pain, the shoulder injuries persisted, causing me to initially question the efficacy of the ABRM. Simple exercises, such as the stationary hang (hanging from a bar to decompress the spine and shoulders), remained excruciating due to the strain on the scarred tendons and muscles, constantly reminding me of my limitations.

I vividly recall a severe incident in my mid-twenties while doing standing shoulder presses with a single fifty-pound dumbbell. While lifting to exhaustion, I briefly lost control of the weight, which yanked my shoulder out of its proper alignment. The pain was paralyzing, leaving that arm unusable for months. The subsequent lack of use led to dramatic muscle wasting due to atrophy. To rehabilitate it, I had to approach the recovery process not only by applying the ABR Maneuvers for the first time to this specific joint but by obsessively studying shoulder anatomy to properly figure out how to put its functionality back together.

Recovery as an Active Exploration

Recovery is not a passive waiting game; it is an active process requiring you to take the initiative to find and address the precise sources of your pain and dysfunction. Just because your shoulder feels fine in a neutral resting position does not mean you are free from injury or underlying weakness. Engaging in targeted exercises and exploring various ranges of motion are crucial for uncovering hidden vulnerabilities in your musculature and identifying deep trigger points.

This proactive approach strengthens your body, your resolve, and your self-confidence. Now, if I experience a flare-up or a minor injury to my shoulder or almost anywhere else, I can usually remove the pain the same day by applying the ABRM. The journey to overcoming shoulder pain is not merely about alleviating discomfort; it is about rediscovering your strength and embracing a healthier, more resilient self.

Fun Fact: The rotator cuff muscles, which are key stabilizers of the shoulder, are anatomically designed to act more like brakes than accelerators. They primarily function to slow down and stabilize the joint during fast movements, which is why tears often happen when throwing or catching, due to failed deceleration.

Chapter Fourteen

The Secret Language of Your Hands: Why They Hold Your Body's Stress

O ur hands are arguably the most remarkable tools the human body possesses. They are the instruments through which we create, communicate, and connect with the world, boasting an intricate complexity that few other body parts can match. Yet, this constant, necessary activity—from the moment we wake until we sleep, typing, gripping, and lifting—comes at a cost. The hands are prone to accumulating stress and deep tension due to their incessant use. This chapter explores how the Autonomic Bio Recovery Maneuvers (ABRM) can help you systematically target and release this accumulated pain, allowing you to not only alleviate discomfort but to rediscover the innate power of muscle memory.

The hands, fingers, and thumbs are the most heavily used and, consequently, the most stressed parts of the body. This continuous, low-grade use takes a significant toll, causing stress and tension to accumulate in the intricate network of muscles, tendons, and ligaments. This results in common ailments like stiffness, reduced dexterity, and chronic conditions like Carpal Tunnel Syndrome. However, the issue transcends simple physical discomfort. The hands are a crucial extension of the nervous system, meaning that accumulated stress in the hands can directly mirror and amplify stress in the mind and the rest of the body. This physical tension is often a direct neurological bottleneck.

Muscle memory is an incredible neurological mechanism that allows us to perform complex tasks—such as playing a musical instrument or typing—without conscious thought. It relies on repetitive practice to "hardwire" movements into the brain and muscles. Unfortunately, this very mechanism can work against us. Over time, poor posture, habitual clenching, and restricted movement caused by stress and tension can become equally "hardwired" into the hand muscles. The ABRM helps reverse these maladaptive patterns by releasing chronic tension, restoring natural flexibility, and reconnecting the hand's natural range of motion to the central nervous system. Stress on the hands stems not just from simple overuse but from the repetitive, often unnatural motions demanded by modern life, such as constant screen swiping, gripping a smartphone, or continuous typing. This strain leads to specific functional imbalances, including tightness in the palms and fingers from chronic gripping, weakness in the thumbs from device overuse, and imbalanced strength where the dominant hand carries more tension. This constant strain can even lead to nerve compression, causing pain, tingling, or numbness that radiates up the arm, known as neuropathy.

The Autonomic Bio Recovery Maneuvers provide a practical, targeted approach to releasing this tension and restoring functionality to the hands. This is an active self-healing process that begins with Somatic Awareness: observing your hands at rest and during movement to identify areas of chronic stiffness. Next, you Target the Tension Points by using the opposite hand, a massage tool, or a small ball to apply firm but gentle pressure to key tension reservoirs: the base of the thumb (thenar eminence), the center of the palm, and the pads of the fingers. Press firmly, hold for a count of five, and release slowly to initiate neurological change. Following this, you must Activate and Mobilize the muscles by slowly opening and closing your hands and spreading your fingers wide to restore circulation and full range of motion. Finally, Integrate Respiratory Control by using deep, measured breathing (inhaling as you spread your fingers and exhaling as you curl them into a fist) to directly relax the autonomic nervous system, enhancing the ABRM's effect.

The results of using the ABRM on your hands are often immediate and surprisingly far-reaching. You will experience Improved Dexterity, Enhanced Circulation (which aids in micro-degradation reversal), and a profound sense of Stress Relief as physical tension in the hands relaxes the central nervous system. This process helps you Reestablish Muscle Memory for effortless, fluid movements. Furthermore, healing the hands provides secondary benefits that impact the entire body: Sharper Mental Focus (due to the dense sensory-motor connection between hands and the brain); Better Posture (by relieving strain that travels up the wrists and forearms to the shoulders); and a sense of Emotional Release, as the hands are highly expressive and can harbor physical manifestations of psychological stress. Investing in the longevity and functionality of your hands with the ABRM is an investment in your entire self, allowing you to experience the freedom of having fully functional, pain-free hands. The hands, fingers, and thumbs are your body's most used—and most stressed—parts. Yet they hold incredible potential for renewal and vitality. By applying the ABRM, you can release the buildup of stress and tension, rediscover the memory of muscle memory, and experience the freedom of having fully functional, pain-free hands. Your hands are your connection to the world. Take care of them, and they will continue to serve you in truly extraordinary ways.

Fun Fact: The complex mechanics of the hand require 34 muscles (18 in the forearm and 16 in the hand) and 27 bones just to operate the five fingers. This immense density of required movement and control is why chronic stress quickly accumulates and why focused relief is so effective.

CHAPTER FIFTEEN

THE ENGINE OF VITALITY: HOW TO COMMAND YOUR HEART AND LUNGS

Your heart and lungs are the tireless engines of your vitality, working every second of every day to sustain life. Yet, over time, these vital systems can become burdened by a subtle buildup of cellular waste, chronic inflammation, and physical stress. In this chapter, I will explain how the Autonomic Bio Recovery Method (ABRM) offers a unique, non-invasive way to take control of these processes, helping you eliminate accumulated stagnation and experience incredible side effects, including renewed energy, youthfulness, and profound vitality.

A core principle of the ABRM is: "You cannot clean and recover what you cannot control." This concept applies directly to the complex network of muscles and tissues surrounding your heart and lungs. When these support muscles—including the diaphragm, intercostals, and deep postural stabilizers—are underdeveloped or atrophied, they lose their ability to function correctly. This dysfunction doesn't just reduce efficiency; it contributes to tissue breakdown, localized inflammation, and systemic weakness. Inflammation is particularly dangerous when it affects the musculature connected to the heart, as a weak, clogged system can suffer, potentially leading to severe conditions. Our bodies accumulate waste from various sources, including environmental toxins, dust, and fat deposits; this buildup can clog the arteries, burden the lungs, and weaken the heart. Factors like smoking or exposure to pollutants accelerate this issue, creating stubborn internal buildup that compromises the body's essential efficiency.

This internal buildup is not limited to the cardiovascular system; undigested food and waste create inflammation, blockages, and systemic stress in the gastrointestinal (GI) system as well. This GI stagnation often mirrors the accumulation seen in the cardiovascular and respiratory systems, highlighting the body's interconnected nature. The key to rejuvenation is to actively activate and cleanse these systems to restore their full functional capacity. The ABRM offers a unique approach that activates the specific muscles and tissues connected to these vital organs, significantly improving their mechanical function and aiding in the clearance of accumulated waste.

You can stimulate and cleanse your heart and lungs by integrating the ABRM with proven physical actions. The three main methods are: 1. Exercise: Physical activity naturally forces your heart to pump harder and your lungs to expand fully, improving circulation, clearing out stagnant blood, and maximizing tissue oxygenation. 2. Breathing Exercises: Controlled, deep diaphragmatic breathing not only strengthens the lungs themselves but also mechanically massages the heart and surrounding muscles (the intercostals and diaphragm). This process releases stored, chronic tension and improves cardio-respiratory efficiency. 3. Targeted ABRM Techniques: By focusing on the muscles that attach to the rib cage and extend to and from the heart (such as the chest, diaphragm, and intercostal muscles), you can directly influence the mechanical function of your cardiovascular and respiratory systems. Using ABRM, you stimulate these muscles to neurologically release tension, which enhances circulation and oxygen exchange efficiency, effectively helping the body expel waste.

When you effectively engage these vital systems using the ABRM, the results are immediate and transformative: you achieve Improved Circulation, as blood flows more freely, carrying oxygen and nutrients more efficiently; you facilitate the Clearing Out of Toxins, as stagnant waste stored in chronic tension points is released; and you experience Increased Energy, as your now-efficient heart and lungs make you feel younger and less fatigued. Crucially, your Restored Confidence allows the fear of physical exertion to disappear as your body begins to function with its intended capability. The buildup in your body is not just about what you ingest; it is also about what your body fails to process and eliminate, such as fatty deposits and potential arterial plaque. The ABRM works by activating and strengthening the muscles that support these systems, helping your body expel this residual waste. For instance, stimulating the diaphragm and intercostal muscles enhances lung function, allowing for deeper, more effective breathing, which, in turn, enhances the body's systemic oxygen saturation.

When you apply the ABRM to your heart, lungs, and surrounding muscles, the side effects are truly remarkable. You will notice Renewed Youthfulness, feeling as though you have turned back the clock; Enhanced Physical Performance, where once-exhausting activities become effortless; Sharper Mental Clarity, as improved oxygen flow benefits the brain, reducing brain fog; and often, a powerful Emotional Release linked to the cleansing of these stressed systems. The Autonomic Bio Recovery System is not merely about pain relief or waste removal; it is about rediscovering the energy and vitality that has always resided within you. By taking proactive control of your most vital systems, you unlock a better, stronger, more energetic version of yourself.

Fun Fact: The average adult human at rest takes between 12 and 20 breaths per minute. Using deep, diaphragmatic breathing (a technique promoted by the ABRM) can lower this rate to as little as 6 breaths per minute, signaling the Autonomic Nervous System to shift from a high-stress "fight-or-flight" state to a deep, healing "rest-and-digest" state.

Chapter Sixteen

BEYOND PAIN RELIEF: WHY EXERCISE IS THE ANCHOR OF THE ROBERTS METHOD

If you've ever fixed a car's engine only to leave the body to rust, you understand the core principle of this chapter: the Roberts Method is the neurological fix, but regular exercise is the necessary structural maintenance. The methodologies and techniques outlined in this book, while powerful for pain removal, must be combined with a structured exercise program. My approach is a wellness technique and an alternative pain management strategy designed to alleviate muscle discomfort, but it is absolutely crucial to understand that using the ABR Maneuvers *alone* may prevent the pain from truly being permanent. Regular exercise is the non-negotiable key component in preventing pain recurrence, as it helps to rebuild lost muscle strength, enhance physical resilience, and improve essential support for the affected areas. This synergistic, holistic approach significantly diminishes the likelihood of pain re-emerging.

The "Use It or Lose It" Principle and Micro-Degradation

The risk of relying solely on the ABR Method for pain relief is high; if you neglect to engage in any form of strengthening exercise afterward, the pain is highly likely to return. As discussed in the chapter on aging, the principle of micro-degradation succinctly illustrates the concept of "use it or lose it." Pain removal with the ABRM *opens the door* to function, but only deliberate physical activity steps through it. Regular physical activity—such as walking, swimming, weightlifting, yoga, and other sports—is fundamental for maintaining muscle mass, bone density, and overall functionality, especially as we advance in years. The combination of the ABRM with exercise offers a unique opportunity to potentially recover some muscle strength and coordination that has been lost due to years of compensatory movement, thereby promoting a sustainable and active lifestyle.

Designing Your Integrated Exercise Program

What type of exercise is recommended? The ideal approach involves a consistent regimen of light to moderate physical activity. This should include a balance of key components: cardiovascular work (like walking or swimming), strength training (like light weightlifting or resistance exercises), and dedicated stretching or flexibility work (like yoga or Pilates). Incorporating a variety of activities is essential; it not only keeps the regimen engaging but ensures that diverse muscle groups are activated, fostering holistic strength and flexibility throughout the body. Monitoring your body for discomfort and pain during these activities is paramount—this continuous, mindful awareness will drive improvement and prevent re-injury.

To maximize the benefits of the ABRM's recalibration, integrating strength training with cardiovascular exercises is vital. Strength training is essential for maintaining muscle mass and bone density, which are critical health markers, while cardiovascular activities promote heart health and improve endurance. Flexibility and balance exercises, such as yoga or Pilates, further enhance your range of motion and drastically reduce the risk of age-related falls.

The Mind-Body Connection and "Optimal Performance"

Beyond the physical benefits, incorporating the ABR Maneuvers with regular exercise nurtures a powerful positive mind-body connection. Exercise releases endorphins, the body's natural pain-relieving chemicals, which enhance mood and reduce stress. This effect perfectly complements the physical pain-relief aspects of my technique, fostering a deep sense of well-being and empowering you to take proactive control of your health journey. While this process may make you feel like you are "aging backward," it's important to understand this feeling as striving for optimal performance for your current age and physical condition. The aim is to approach your personal best, free from injury and with muscles in peak condition. As you reclaim lost capabilities, that sense of recovery naturally evokes the energy of youth.

This emphasis on regaining abilities and even acquiring new skills is vital. Many individuals, especially those who suffered chronic pain from a young age, may never have been able to safely engage in certain activities. By adopting this integrated approach, you can explore new avenues for personal growth and development, fostering a profound sense of accomplishment and inspiration. In conclusion, combining the Roberts Method with a well-rounded exercise program creates a synergistic approach to pain management, muscle recovery, and overall wellness that addresses physical limitations while promoting a more fulfilling and active life.

Fun Fact: Sarcopenia, the age-related loss of muscle mass, is so significant that the average person can lose approximately 3% to 8% of their muscle mass per decade after the age of 30. This process is the primary reason why combining nerve-based recovery (ABRM) with resistance exercise is critical for graceful aging.

Chapter Seventeen

GRIT, RESILIENCE, AND THE RELENTLESS PURSUIT OF HEALING

The foundational work that led to the development of the **Autonomic Bio Recovery (ABR) Maneuvers** was a deeply personal and solitary endeavor, positioning the developer simultaneously as the patient and the doctor, the experiment and the researcher, and the sufferer determined to solve their own agony. When this arduous journey began, there was no pre-existing map or instruction manual to follow; the path was shrouded in darkness and defined by the relentless presence of pain. Consequently, every breakthrough, every principle, and every maneuver detailed in the ABR method was laboriously discovered through a grueling process of **trial and error**, sustained persistence, profound frustration, and an unwavering belief in the possibility of healing. This was not a method that was passively received; it was painstakingly *carved* out of the severe suffering that defined daily life. The ABR Maneuvers were truly born from the absolute necessity of finding a solution, from enduring chronic suffering, and, most crucially, from an absolute refusal to accept that pain would forever dictate the terms of existence.

The severity of the challenge presented constant opportunities to surrender, and under normal circumstances, many people would have. Pain is a formidable antagonist; it not only inflicts physical devastation but also launches a corrosive attack on one's **confidence**, motivation, and fundamental belief in a functional future. Yet, an inner resolve—a stubborn refusal to capitulate—provided the driving force. Every physical setback became an unexpected lesson, forcing the developer to engage in deep learning about the subtle yet profound ways the body communicates its distress and its path toward healing. Every moment of failure was not a dead end, but an essential piece of the puzzle that slowly began to form a coherent picture of neurological and mechanical compensation. This journey demanded a quality known as **grit**—not the superficial variety quoted on a wall, but the deeply forged resolve that develops when one's back is against the wall, when all initial plans have failed, and when exhaustion, pain, and overwhelming odds persist. Grit is fundamentally the choice to take the next step when no one is observing, when results are painfully slow, and when the process is seemingly incomprehensible to outsiders.

The quality of **resilience** was the essential fuel that ensured forward movement, enabling the continuous confrontation of fear, frustration, and debilitating uncertainty without allowing these forces to completely derail progress. Resilience is not defined by the absence of fear, but by the certainty of getting back up every single time one falls. It requires a deep-seated trust that the difficult process is actively shaping and strengthening the individual, even during the most painful moments of struggle. The ABR method was conceptualized in the dark and is now shared in the light, carrying the message that true healing is holistic—it is a transformation that is physical, mental, emotional, and spiritual. The recovery process is not just about restoring functional capacity to the body; it is fundamentally about recovering one's **belief in self**. The profound lesson gleaned from this struggle is simple: your pain is a temporary state, not your permanent identity; your setback is information, not your definitive ending; and your challenges should be viewed not as impassable barriers, but as invitations to evolve. Every goal, every dream, and every major breakthrough begins with that single, resolute choice: the choice **not to quit**.

The path to recovery often remains unknown and unclear. Just like the developer, one must begin with the resources at hand, starting exactly where they are, and committing to taking one step, then another, and then another. Progress is often deceptively invisible for long periods, until suddenly it becomes undeniably clear. **Leadership begins with leading oneself**; if a person can relentlessly refuse to quit on their own healing, that determination will inevitably translate into success in all other aspects of their life and dreams. The ABR Method's profound impact extends far beyond mere physical correction; it actively reshaped the developer's understanding of self. It underscored the truth that every obstacle contains critical information, every struggle holds wisdom, and every challenge is pregnant with untapped potential. Crucially, the greatest, most transformative breakthroughs often occur immediately after the precise moment when the temptation to give up was at its strongest. The journey of healing is continuous, but the commitment to keep going, to keep leaning forward, and to keep refusing to be defeated is what transforms suffering into discovery, and discovery into profound, lasting transformation.

Fun Fact: The concept of **Grit** as a psychological trait, championed by psychologist Angela Duckworth, is often measured by a person's sustained interest and effort toward long-term goals. Her research found that grit is a **better predictor of success** in many challenging endeavors (like academic achievement or professional pursuits) than traditional measures like IQ or talent.

Chapter Eighteen

Empowered Healing: The Role of Self-Reliance and Self-Care in Pain Management

S elf-reliance is one of the most powerful tools for overcoming pain and restoring health. The idea of taking charge of your healing process can be both empowering and transformative. This chapter examines the significance of self-reliance and self-care in managing pain, and how these principles can augment the effectiveness of the Roberts Method and the Autonomic Bio Recovery Maneuvers. We will delve into concepts such as personal responsibility, proactive health management, mindfulness, and the psychology of healing, all of which play crucial roles in achieving a pain-free life and maintaining long-term well-being.

Self-reliance is more than just a mindset; it is a call to action that challenges individuals to take ownership of their health. When faced with chronic pain or injury, many people feel powerless and dependent on external interventions, be it medications, surgeries, or other treatments. However, self-reliance in healing promotes a shift from dependency to autonomy. By adopting a self-reliant approach, you actively take part in your recovery journey. This does not mean rejecting medical advice or professional help but supplementing it with your knowledge and efforts. The Click It Out method is a prime example of how self-reliance can be applied. Instead of waiting for external solutions, you learn to listen to your body, understand its signals, and engage in techniques that address pain at its source.

Self-reliance empowers you to experiment, adjust, and refine your pain management strategies based on your unique experiences and needs. It is about cultivating the belief that you can have a significant impact on your well-being. This belief catalyzes change, encouraging you to take the steps necessary to reclaim your body and life from pain.

Self-care goes together with self-reliance. It involves deliberately nurturing your physical, mental, and emotional health. In pain management, self-care is not just about temporary relief but also about fostering a holistic environment where the body can heal and thrive. Core elements of self-care that can be integrated into your daily life to support the Roberts Method:

1. Mindful Movement: Gentle exercises and stretching can help maintain flexibility and balance your muscles. These movements can prevent muscle compensation, promote circulation, and reduce inflammation, complementing your self-adjustment efforts.

2. Nutrition: Proper nutrition fuels the body's healing processes. A diet rich in anti-inflammatory foods, including fruits, vegetables, lean proteins, and healthy fats, supports tissue repair and helps reduce pain.

3. Sleep and Rest: Adequate and quality sleep is crucial for recovery. The body performs much of its repair work during sleep, and disruptions to this process can impair the healing response. Developing good sleep hygiene and managing stress can help improve sleep quality, enhancing recovery.

4. Stress Management: Stress can worsen pain and hinder recovery. Techniques like deep breathing, meditation, or mindfulness can help manage stress levels, creating a more conducive environment for healing.

5. Hydration: Staying well-hydrated is essential for keeping healthy joints, muscles, and overall bodily functions. Water supports cellular processes that are vital for tissue repair and recovery.

A proactive and positive mindset can have a direct impact on pain perception and recovery outcomes. Developing psychological resilience is a part of self-reliance, as it empowers you to face pain challenges head-on and adapt to setbacks. Here's how psychological aspects contribute to healing:

- Belief in Recovery: Believing you can heal is a powerful motivator. A positive outlook can influence the brain's pain regulation mechanisms, reduce pain perception, and enhance the effectiveness of self-adjustment techniques. I feel that it is my strong belief in God that led me to discovery this life changing method.

- Patience and Persistence: Healing needs patience and persistence, mainly when relying on self-care and self-adjustment methods. Understanding that recovery is difficult can help you stay motivated and consistent in your efforts.

- Learning from Pain: Pain is not just a symptom but a signal. Viewing pain as a guide rather than an enemy allows you to learn more about your body's needs and adjust your strategies accordingly. This perspective is crucial in following your "pain path" to complete recovery. It is also important to learn how the body compensates for pain when you become injured.

- Building a Supportive Routine: Creating a routine incorporating self-reliance and self-care is essential for sustainable pain management. Begin with small, manageable changes and gradually develop a comprehensive routine that suits your lifestyle. Consistency is key; even the most effective techniques require regular application to yield lasting results.

- Daily Check-ins: Start each day with a body scan or mindfulness practice to assess your emotional state. Find any areas of tension or discomfort and plan to address them using the ABR Maneuvers.

- Reflect and Adapt: Regularly reflect on your progress. What is working well? What needs adjustment? Self-reliance involves being flexible and open to adjusting your routine to achieve optimal results.

By embracing self-reliance and self-care, you take control of your healing journey. These principles focus on managing pain and promoting a comprehensive approach to health that encourages balance, strength, and resilience. Remember, the path to health is personal, and with self-reliance and self-care as your guides, you can walk it confidently, free from the limitations of pain.

Top of Form

Bottom of Form

CHAPTER NINETEEN

BEYOND PAIN: THE QUIET TRIUMPH OF "BUSINESS AS USUAL"

I f chronic pain is your body yelling for help, then what is true healing? It isn't a flash of light or a ringing bell; it's a profound, quiet shift back to effortless functionality. The process of the Autonomic Bio Recovery Maneuvers (ABRM) offers a personalized, self-directed path to pain management and recovery. This method systematically reduces pain, enhances muscle function, encourages mobility, and promotes a balanced and healthy musculoskeletal system. The key to successful, long-term recovery lies in understanding your body's pain signals and diligently following the path they outline, which is fundamental to achieving sustained health and vitality.

The Critical Phase of Rebuilding Strength

One of the most important things to understand is that when you successfully apply the Autonomic Bio Recovery Maneuvers to remove pain, the affected muscle or connective tissue will not be instantly strong. During this period—the crucial post-release phase—you must remain cautious. The muscle and connective tissue need dedicated time to rebuild strength, much like an ankle sprain or a bone fracture requires rest for structural integration. Overuse, strain, or the resumption of poor posture can easily undo your progress, forcing you to use the ABR Maneuvers again. Furthermore, muscle strain can quickly trigger new compensation patterns in surrounding muscle groups, causing new imbalances or unexpected pain in seemingly unrelated areas. Your musculoskeletal system works as a single, interdependent unit. Think of your body like a carefully tuned instrument: if you break one string, the entire composition changes. The ABRM fixes the string, but you must allow time for the instrument to be played gently before resuming a full performance.

The Silence of Full Recovery

There is a powerful moment in the healing process that many people miss because it is entirely silent. When you are injured, your body speaks loudly and unmistakably: the pain is a constant, persistent signal from your nervous system yelling, "There is a problem here. Pay attention!" You don't have to guess when something is wrong. But when your body is fully healed, there is no grand announcement. There is no alert or celebratory sensation. The once-injured area doesn't say, "Hey, just letting you know—I'm good now." Instead, something more subtle—and more powerful—happens: the area simply goes back to work. Quietly. Naturally. Without needing your conscious attention.

This is what I call the state of "business as usual." The limb moves without resistance; the joint functions without effort. The muscle no longer calls for help. You become unaware of the area—not because it doesn't matter, but because it is no longer in crisis. This silence is how your body truly signals full recovery. Many people miss this distinction. When a body part truly returns to its baseline, it doesn't keep asking for help—it just gets back to its job. With the Autonomic Bio Recovery Method, the goal is not just temporary pain reduction, it is to guide the body back to a state where the nervous system stops sending distress signals entirely. If you re-injure an area, you will have to apply the ABR Maneuvers again. As you recover, treat the healing period with respect; let the nervous system stabilize and let the muscle reestablish its role. However, there are times when the ABR Maneuvers can only be used for pain management. For instance, in my case, where I have arthritis in my spinal discs, the discs will never fully recover, but I can always rely on the ABR Maneuvers to manage and eliminate acute pain symptoms.

Thank you for allowing me to share this journey with you. The power to achieve "business as usual" is now in your hands. Through consistency and dedication, the ABRM can help you unlock the true potential of your body.

Fun Fact: The nerve cells responsible for detecting pain, called nociceptors, only account for less than 1% of all sensory receptors in the human body, yet they are wired so efficiently that their signals immediately bypass many sensory filters to ensure you react instantly to injury.

BACK COVER

F or millions, chronic pain is more than discomfort—it's a daily prison. Medications, surgeries, and traditional therapies often provide only temporary relief, leaving people searching for answers.

The Chronic Pain Cure introduces the groundbreaking **Autonomic Bio Recovery Method (ABRM)**, a revolutionary approach that doesn't mask pain, but addresses its root source within the nervous system and muscles. Developed through years of struggle, discovery, and perseverance, this method offers a natural, repeatable, and life-changing way to eliminate pain and restore vitality.

Inside, you'll learn:

- Why pain is more than a symptom—and how it signals hidden dysfunction.

- Step-by-step techniques to release pain from any muscle in the body.

- How to restore clarity, improve recovery, and activate the body's natural resilience.

- Practical guidance to regain control over your health, energy, and mindset.

This is not another quick fix—it's a complete system designed to empower you to live pain-free, regain confidence, and reclaim the life you thought was lost.

9 798992 361148